Successful Qualitative Health Research

Successful Qualitative Health Research

A practical introduction

Emily C. Hansen

Open University Press

Open University Press
McGraw-Hill Education
McGraw-Hill House
Shoppenhangers Road
Maidenhead
Berkshire
England
SL6 2QL

email: enquiries@openup.co.uk
world wide web: www.openup.co.uk

and Two Penn Plaza, New York, NY 10121-2289, USA

First published 2006

A catalogue record of this book is available from the British Library

ISBN-10: 0 335 22034 7 (pb) 0 335 22035 5 (hb)
ISBN-13: 9780 335 220342 (pb) 9780 335 220359 (hb)

Library of Congress Cataloging-in-Publication Data
CIP data applied for

Typeset by Midland Typesetters, Australia
Printed by South Wind Production, Singapore

CONTENTS

PREFACE

There has been an increase in the application and status of qualitative research in health-related fields (Dixon-Woods & Fitzpatrick 2001; Thomas, J. et al. 2004). People working or studying in health-related fields are realising that a familiarity with qualitative research methods is a useful skill to acquire. The growth in qualitative research has occurred as research and evaluation have become a more important part of everyday life for people studying or working in health-related fields. Government programs are encouraging students, medical practitioners, allied health professionals, policy makers and consumers to conduct and use research and evaluation more. Understanding how research is conducted and the principles underpinning different research designs allows healthcare practitioners and policy makers to critically appraise research evidence, to apply research findings appropriately, to identify issues or problems that require additional research and to conduct research for themselves.

There is also a shift occurring in the types of research being conducted in the health sphere. There has been rapid growth in the perceived importance of consumer views about health and healthcare, and of health services research focused on the ways that people use services and how services can be improved. Furthermore, collaborative and multidisciplinary research teams are increasingly seen as desirable for conducting research. Research teams often include researchers from diverse backgrounds, including the social sciences, nursing and allied health (Lambert & McKevitt 2002; Creswell 2003). Each researcher brings expertise and awareness of research methods and methodologies from their own disciplinary backgrounds so that the teams span a wide range, collectively. There is a consequent need for researchers in health to develop skills in qualitative research and to familiarise themselves with the qualitative research approach:

> Qualitative research claims to describe lifeworlds 'from the inside out', from the point of view of the people who participate. By so doing it seeks to contribute to a better understanding of social realities and to draw attention to processes, meanings, patterns and structural features. (Flick et al. 2004:3)

In my capacity as a teacher of qualitative research methods, I have found that many new qualitative researchers struggle to produce rigorous qualitative research as a result of their inexperience and lack of formal training. For newcomers, the field of qualitative research is broad, complex and often confusing (Flick et al. 2004:3). Thus when novice qualitative researchers try to find advice in the form of textbooks, they may feel overwhelmed by the volume and complexity of the literature. Those who are already practising in health-related professions and those currently training in health-related fields are often at a particular disadvantage when they try to learn about qualitative research because qualitative research differs considerably from the scientific medical research paradigm with which they are most familiar (Morse & Field 1996:18).

Successful Qualitative Health Research is aimed at the ever-growing numbers of researchers in health who require a user-friendly book containing practical and theoretical advice about conducting qualitative research. It provides the reader with advice about designing a research project utilising qualitative methods, collecting different types of qualitative data and what to do with this data once it is collected (i.e. analysis and presentation). Unlike many other texts about applied qualitative research, this book also contains detailed descriptions of different methods of data analysis plus advice on writing up qualitative research. Furthermore, as qualitative data analysis techniques have a rich theoretical history and are marked by ongoing debate, each chapter of the book provides the reader with background information about the ideas and arguments underpinning the methods discussed in that chapter. Related to this, I have referred to foundational qualitative research texts and studies as well as to newer studies throughout the book. Qualitative research as we use it today owes a great deal to sociological and anthropological research and writing produced in the 1960s, '70s and '80s. Thus, unlike many other textbooks in health that reference only the latest studies, this book attempts to give the reader a sense of the history and social context of contemporary qualitative research.

Five chapters also feature 'real life' case study examples of qualitative research written by experienced researchers from health-related disciplines including public health, nursing, health program evaluation and sociology. The case studies are inspiring for beginning researchers and should provide the reader with new ideas and a feeling for the wide range of opportunities offered by qualitative research. With these inputs, *Successful Qualitative Health Research* sits in a middle ground between basic 'recipe book' style approaches and the more complex and abstract style of writing and discussion found in textbooks designed for an advanced academic audience.

ACKNOWLEDGMENTS

I owe thanks to a large number of people who assisted, supported and advised me while I was writing this book. These people include all of the case study authors, plus Peter Mudge, Steve Lockwood, Andrew Robinson, Hazel Easthope, Suzanne McNeill, Clarissa Cook, Chris Easthope, Roberta Julian, Gary Easthope and other staff members and students at the School of Sociology and Social Work and the Discipline of General Practice at the University of Tasmania. Jane Lambert provided considerable assistance with editing and formatting the manuscript.

Comments from anonymous reviewers were extremely helpful and encouraging. I would like to express my appreciation for the way they engaged with the material and the suggestions they made for its improvement.

My thanks also go to Elizabeth Weiss, Emma Cant, Emma Sorensen, Colette Vella, Joanne Holliman and Anne Reilly at Allen & Unwin for their assistance and encouragement.

Finally, the book could not have been completed without salary support from the Australian Commonwealth Department of Health and Ageing via the Primary Healthcare Research Evaluation and Development Strategy (PHCRED).

one

QUALITATIVE RESEARCH: AN INTRODUCTION

Qualitative research is becoming increasingly respected and popular among health researchers (Thomas, J. et al. 2004). This is because qualitative research methods are well suited for investigating the meanings, interpretations, social and cultural norms and perceptions that impact on health-related behaviour, medical practice and health outcomes (Jordens & Little 2004; Sayre 2000). They also allow researchers to explore issues from the perspectives of the individuals directly involved; for example, the experiences of spousal carers of people with multiple sclerosis, and the disclosure strategies used by adults with cystic fibrosis (Cheung & Hocking 2004; Lowton 2004).

This chapter provides an introduction to research as an activity and to qualitative research in particular. It presents the differences between qualitative and quantitative research, discusses combining qualitative and quantitative research and explains the close relationship between qualitative research and academic theory. The chapter provides essential background material for the following chapters in this book.

Defining research

Many people seem unsure about what research actually is. Popular conceptions of research often imply that it is rather mysterious, esoteric and invariably difficult. While research certainly can be all of these things, it doesn't have to be. In fact, it can be an enjoyable and satisfying activity with the potential to improve healthcare practice, planning and policy.

Because it is much easier to do something successfully if you understand what it is you are trying to achieve, I decided to start this book with a brief discussion about the meaning of research.

There are many different types of research and, on the surface, these may vary considerably. For example, compare a scientist culturing cells in a laboratory, an epidemiologist collecting information about bone mineral density in pre-menopausal women, an anthropologist living in a South American village and a social worker running focus groups with young mothers to learn about their needs. All of these people are conducting research if their inquiry meets the following criteria. First, for an inquiry to be called research, it should involve a disciplined and systematic search for knowledge. A researcher uses systematic, clearly described procedures; they are aware of the strengths and weaknesses of these methods; they value empirical verification; and seek plausible alternative explanations for their findings (Smith & Glass 1987:11).

Second, for an inquiry to be research, it should be a public activity available for scrutiny by peers. This involves clearly describing how the new knowledge was achieved and disseminating research results. For the majority of health-related research, this scrutiny will also involve review of a research proposal or protocol by an ethics committee or institutional research review board before the research is conducted.

A third and closely related characteristic of research is that it is an activity that should not occur in isolation. Research is 'original creative intellectual activity leading to the generation of new knowledge' (Whitworth 1994:26). The work of individual researchers is viewed as part of a larger process of finding answers. Associated with this is an expectation that the outcomes of research (including knowledge gained about methods and approaches) should be in some way transferable to other researchers and make a contribution to wider stocks of knowledge; for example, producing new information, testing existing knowledge or finding new applications for existing knowledge (Pryke et al. 2003).

Types of research

There are a number of different types of research relevant to the readers of this book. The first of these is social research. Social research refers to any research that investigates human behaviours and social life (Berg 2004). All qualitative research is social research; however, not all social research is qualitative research. The methods used by social researchers are largely derived from a group of academic disciplines known collectively as the social sciences. These include sociology, anthropology, education, psychology, geography and political science.

Other types of research may be defined by the purpose of the inquiry – descriptive research, explanatory research and applied research. Descriptive and explanatory research are undertaken because the researcher wants to contribute to the stock of knowledge and has interest and expertise in a particular field. These types of research tend to be the domain of academic researchers, university students and the occasional individual or group motivated by an overwhelming passion or interest in a particular issue or problem. In contrast, applied research is 'specifically designed to be problem solving and to have an outcome which is expected to be of immediate relevance' (Macoun 2004:1; Royse et al. 2001:2). Applied research is conducted because the researchers want to gain knowledge in order to meet a need, solve a problem or achieve a commercial objective. A wide range of people in addition to academics and students carry out applied social research. These include professional and market researchers, healthcare practitioners, educators, policy makers and managers. Evaluation research conducted to determine the success of programs can be seen as a type of applied research (Royse et al. 2001:2).

Evaluation provides information about the processes and outcomes of health-related programs for use by those involved in planning, implementing and funding them (Smith & Glass 1987:30). 'Social programs, and the policies that spawn and justify them, aim to improve the welfare of individuals, organisations and society. Hence, it is useful to assess how much any social program improves welfare, how it does so and how can it do so more effectively' (Shadish et al. 1991:19). Evaluation research can be undertaken during a program to assess implementation and at the conclusion of a program to assess how well the program met specified objectives. For example, while descriptive and explanatory research might produce results that suggest a relationship between vaccination rates and the incidence of childhood disease, the ensuing vaccination program can be evaluated to assess issues such as cost effectiveness, uptake and sustainability (House 1980:121). As with other aspects of health-related research, evaluation practitioners are increasingly making use of qualitative methods and approaches (Owen 1999; Burgess 1991; Patton 1990).

> Qualitative methods permit the evaluator to study selected issues in depth and detail. Approaching fieldwork without being constrained by predetermined categories of analysis contributes to the depth, openness and detail of qualitative inquiry. (Patton 1990:13)

Establishing whether the social research you plan to conduct is applied, descriptive or explanatory is your first step. It will impact on how the

3

research is conducted, and expectations about research dissemination and outcomes.

Qualitative research

In qualitative research, behaviours, understandings, actions and experiences are not measured using statistical analysis as in quantitative research (Devers 1999; Sofaer 1999). Instead, detailed written descriptions and explanations of the phenomena under investigation are produced. Baum describes this difference by stating that: 'quantitative research attempts to reduce and measure social phenomena while qualitative research aims to understand social processes' (Baum 1992:1). Qualitative methods are those that collect data in the form of talk, words, observations, visual images and documents.

Qualitative research is the subject of a longstanding debate among social researchers. From one side of this argument, researchers and writers have claimed that 'social life does not lend itself to any kind of scientific investigation' (Blaikie 1993:2; Smith & Glass 1987:1). Researching how people experience their lives and the meanings and interpretations they give to these aspects is viewed as being fundamentally different from conducting research on natural phenomena or 'things'. Researchers with this viewpoint reject the use of 'scientific method' when investigating the social world, choosing to use an alternative approach often described as constructivist/interpretivist (sometimes also called the inductive paradigm or naturalistic research). Underpinning this approach is the assumption that there is no single reality or truth. From this perspective, research is about discovery arising from active participation by the researcher. 'Hypotheses and theories are generated but the aim of the research is not to prove them to be true or false' (Hamberg et al. 1994:177). Instead, it is assumed that there are a range of possible perceptions of reality and these will change over time and according to social context. In other words, what we are able to know is contextual and situational.

However, proponents of the other side of the argument have insisted that 'there is no aspect of the social world that is not amenable to the application of the scientific method, or at least some kind of scientific method' (Blaikie 1993:3). From this viewpoint (sometimes described as positivist) it is argued that social research should be conducted similarly to other types of scientific research. Studies should be based around hypothesis-testing designs, using statistical analysis and evaluated using criteria such as objectivity, generalisability, validity and reliability (Smith

& Glass 1987:6). Examples are experimental studies or randomised controlled studies using quantitative social research methods such as standardised questionnaires and structured observation.

Most researchers involved in social research fall somewhere between these two positions and tend to use both qualitative and quantitative research methods as they deem appropriate (Sale et al. 2002). However, any researcher using one approach alone or who uses both qualitative and quantitative approaches needs to understand that qualitative and quantitative research are derived from perspectives that assume different views of reality. The two approaches vary in terms of ontology (assumptions about the nature of social reality) and epistemology (assumptions made about how knowledge of reality can be achieved). Many writers argue that qualitative and quantitative research are so dissimilar in their underlying claims and assumptions that they can be seen as representing two different paradigms (Guba & Lincoln 1994:11; Sale et al. 2002; Blaikie 1993). Certainly it is difficult to explain qualitative research without discussing quantitative research as a point of comparison.

Differences between qualitative and quantitative research

Recognising and understanding the differences between qualitative and quantitative research allows a researcher to make informed decisions about the most appropriate approach for their work. It should also assist them to better understand the longstanding historical divide between qualitative and quantitative research (Kelle & Erzberger 2004; Ritchie 2001). The differences between the two approaches are discussed below in terms of underlying assumptions, research design, the research setting and the role of the researcher.

Underlying assumptions

Qualitative research aims to provide 'detailed descriptions and analysis of the quality or substance of the human experience' (Marvasti 2004:7). Qualitative researchers assume that in order to understand human actions and behaviours, we need to understand the meaning and interpretations that people give to their own actions, to the actions of others and to situations and events. Qualitative researchers tend to focus on providing detailed accounts, recognising and explaining social context and discussing ambiguities. A critical stance and explicit questioning of 'taken-for-granted' ways of doing things or assumptions is another common theme found in qualitative research. This includes questioning the assumptions underpinning research methods and theories.

5

Qualitative research encompasses a wide range of theoretical positions. The majority fall within a constructivist/interpretivist paradigm where 'the physical aspects of the world are seen to have independent existence, how the world is perceived (reality) is a social construction' (Martin 1994:7). Preferred methods for learning about the social world are those that emphasise 'human interpretation, inductive reasoning, holistic understanding, qualitative data and contextualised explanation' (Martin 1994:6).

In contrast, quantitative social research derives from a positivist paradigm based on an assumption that the social world can be investigated using scientific method and that there is an independent reality, the 'truth' of which can be found by 'applying the proposition that measurable influences (independent variables) affect measurable outcomes (dependent variables) in a cause–effect manner' (Grbich 1999:15–16). From this perspective it is assumed that 'what is being studied is external to the observer, does not change over time and is not influenced by being observed' (Denzin 1989:24). Reality, truth and facts are viewed as existing externally to the researcher. Quantitative research searches for 'universal explanations for phenomena' (Smith & Glass 1987:23). For example, scientific explanations, if correct, are assumed to apply equally well to all instances of the same problem. Explanation in quantitative research emphasises the quantification of outcomes, generalisability and prediction. This is quite different to the context-based nature of explanations from most qualitative research, where researchers often qualify their statements as applying only to the example under study. Quantitative research tends to have a far more unified theoretical basis than does qualitative research (Martin 1994:3).

Quantitative social research involving the use of statistical measurement is familiar to the majority of people working in the health field. Examples include experimental psychology, standardised health-related quality-of-life questionnaires and large surveys of attitudes and practices. The popularity and widespread use of this type of social research among health researchers reflects the scientific basis of Western medical knowledge and the type of training that most healthcare professionals receive (Martin 1994:3).

Research design

Qualitative research designs can be deductive or inductive. That is, they can aim to test a hypothesis or to develop one (Creswell 2003). However, there is a preference among qualitative researchers for inductive design. While research, by definition, entails the application of disciplined and systematic research methods and study designs, the largely inductive nature of qualitative research projects means that their design tends to alter as the study unfolds in response to changing circumstances and the data being collected (flexibility of design). This is a normal aspect of qualitative research (Denzin & Lincoln 1994).

In contrast, quantitative researchers use standardised and repeatable methodologies that 'represent human experience in numerical categories' (Marvasti 2004:7). These are usually experimental in design (and deductive because they test a pre-existing hypothesis). Experimental design and standardised repeatable methodologies are the cornerstone of quantitative research. Because of this the flexibility of design that characterises the majority of qualitative research is viewed with great suspicion by many quantitative researchers.

Research setting

Qualitative researchers work with data in the form of talk and action that has been collected using methods such as in-depth interviewing, focus groups, observation and textual analysis (Berg 2004). This data is firmly located within its original social context. Consequently, qualitative research is rarely conducted in laboratories or under controlled conditions. Instead, it is conducted in everyday social settings, such as public places, people's homes, workplaces and schools. Some writers refer to qualitative research as 'naturalistic research' in recognition of this feature (Lincoln & Guba 1985; Lofland & Lofland 1984). 'Qualitative data documents the world from the point of view of the people studied . . . rather than presenting it from the point of view of the researcher' (Hammersly 1992:45).

In contrast, quantitative social research is generally conducted in a controlled environment, such as a psychology laboratory, or using anonymous data, such as statistics collected by way of surveys, questionnaires, structured interviews or tests like pulse monitors or x-rays. Due to the requirements of statistical analysis, large amounts of data are often collected. Results are presented in the form of scales, measures and numbers. Because of the types of data collected in quantitative research, the research setting is less important than it is in qualitative research.

Researcher's role

Qualitative researchers try to gather and analyse their own data rather than working with anonymous data collected by other people. They recognise that they are an integral part of the research process.

Their skills, attributes, personal characteristics, interests and views will to some degree impact on the data collected (Morse & Field 1996). It is also common in qualitative research for the researcher to adopt a participatory, collaborative role rather than the objective 'expert' role found in traditional research. Because of their integral role in their research, qualitative researchers try to be 'reflexive'. That is, they attempt to 'engage in explicit, self aware analysis of their own role' (Finlay 2002:531).

However, quantitative researchers adopt a traditional objective/expert role (Martin 1994:7). They attempt to remove their interpretations or prevent them from influencing the research. Accordingly, it is assumed that if the study were repeated using the same methods and study population but different researchers, the results would not vary.

Deciding to use qualitative research

Deciding whether to use a qualitative approach requires careful consideration. The most important factor should be the suitability of the research problem to a qualitative inquiry. However, it is important to critically reflect on the research problem and to take into account how your own views about research may be impacting on your choice.

Many factors have a bearing on a researcher's preferred choice of research approach. While the most important of these should be the usefulness of the approach when addressing a particular research problem, other issues also come into play. What a researcher identifies as an important and 'doable' research problem and how they express this problem will be affected by the ways they view the world and their knowledge of available research approaches. Blaikie (1993:201–2) has identified a number of background issues that may influence a researcher's preference for a particular research approach. These are summarised below:

1 How the approach relates to the world view of the researcher: 'there may be a conscious or unconscious preference for the maintenance of some sort of compatibility between the claims or assumptions that a particular approach makes about the nature of social reality (ontology) and ideological or religious beliefs or values' (Blaikie 1993:201).

2 Personality factors. The choice of a qualitative or a quantitative research strategy 'is likely to be determined by a perceived preference for predetermined, linear procedures as against a perceived ability to manage flexible, ambiguous processes' (Blaikie 1993:201).

3   The professional socialisation of the researcher in terms of disciplinary background (e.g. nursing, medicine, social work, education, sociology, psychology etc) and the institution where the researcher is working. Both of these will influence 'exposure to and experience with particular approaches' (Blaikie 1993:202).
4   The preferences of the audience for the research; for example, the groups or individuals who fund research, the consumers of research, journal editors and journal readers and the research culture of institutions where research is conducted (Blaikie 1993:202).

There are also a number pragmatic issues that researchers need to consider when deciding on the most appropriate research approach to use in a study. 'Certain types of research problems call for specific approaches' (Creswell 2003:21). The following list outlines circumstances when qualitative research is a particularly appropriate choice:

1   Projects where the researcher wants to describe and understand people and to gain insight into how people make sense of their experiences.
2   When the researcher needs a way of understanding issues and relating these to their social context: 'to explain the economic, political, social and cultural factors which influence health and disease; to gain an understanding of how communities and individuals within them interpret health and disease; and to study interactions between the various players who are relevant to any given public health issue' (Baum 1995:464).
3   Exploratory research when the researchers have very little knowledge about an area of investigation and 'where the social contexts of people's lives is of critical significance' (McDonald & Daly 1992:213).
4   When you are trying to gain a new perspective on a problem or issue.
5   Elaboration of causal hypotheses emerging from clinical and epidemiological studies.
6   When you want to conduct research that has relevance and positive meaning for the research participants and where research participants are involved in the research (e.g. action research, community studies).
7   Design issues such as a particularly small study population (i.e. people living with HIV/AIDS in a rural town) and/or when available research funding is tight. Quantitative research generally has to be conducted on a large scale. This can be quite costly. Some qualitative research (while nearly always expensive in terms of time) can be conducted with little more than a researcher, a pen and a notebook.
8   Projects where cases require individual attention because generalising will not give an accurate picture of a situation (Patton 1990:15).

9   Unstable or changeable situations where the flexibility of qualitative research is an advantage.

Many problems can be addressed with either quantitative or qualitative approaches, depending on the specific focus of the study and the ways in which the research problem is expressed. An important aspect of research design is justifying the choices of approach and methods. Both of the above lists contain points that will be helpful when justifying a decision to use qualitative research.

Combining qualitative and quantitative research

Qualitative research is a robust and comprehensive approach with many benefits and strengths. The most common type of qualitative research studies have qualitative methods as the stand-alone research design. The following chapters in this book describe a range of different qualitative methodologies, methods and analytic approaches.

Many research problems are best suited to a purely qualitative inquiry. However, projects that combine the qualitative and quantitative approaches appear to be growing in popularity in the health field (Caracelli & Greene 1993; Casebeer & Verhoef 1997; House 1994). Combining the approaches is sometimes described as mixed methods research. More of this type of research design is being seen in published research, and numerous new books and researcher guides are appearing to assist researchers wanting to conduct mixed methods research (*see* Creswell 2003; Hammersley 1993; Mark & Shortland 1987). The main advantage in combining qualitative and quantitative research in the same project is the increased scope made possible. In some studies a quantitative phase will follow an exploratory qualitative phase. For example, a qualitative study can provide insight into language usage that is helpful when designing a questionnaire. Other studies utilise both approaches in order to 'capture the best of both quantitative and qualitative approaches' (Kushman 1992; Tashakkori & Teddlie 2003). When adopting a mixed methods research design, researchers are able to investigate many different aspects of their research problem. To give a hypothetical example, let's say that a research team investigating increased rates of cigarette smoking among young women has decided that a mixed methods approach will be useful. Their mixed methods study involves the following:

•   In-depth interviews with a range of young women. These will facilitate in-depth one-on-one discussion.

- Focus groups with young women. These will enable researchers to listen to young women talking with each other about smoking.
- A documentary analysis focusing on key texts identified by the participants in the focus groups and interviews, such as magazines, films and television shows watched by young women. This will allow the researchers to see how cigarettes are being portrayed in the popular media and to investigate discourses around cigarette smoking.
- A questionnaire administered to 1500 young women to measure attitudes and self-reported behaviours related to smoking. Questions for the questionnaire would be developed after the qualitative data had been analysed. A questionnaire administered to a large sample allows for generalised statements to be made about attitudes and self-reported behaviours. The use of exploratory qualitative research to develop the questionnaire will increase the validity of the questionnaire data.

As you can see in the above example, utilising a range of research methods and combining qualitative and quantitative research in the same project allows for a detailed and comprehensive inquiry. However, multi-method research designs are not without their problems or critics (Blaikie 1993; Guba 1990). Despite the potential advantages arising from mixed methods studies, everything becomes much more complicated in projects where a number of different data collection methods or data analysis approaches are being used. The epistemological and ontological differences between qualitative and quantitative research will inevitably produce contradictions and ambiguities (Burgess 1993:105). This makes for a more challenging research process and requires a more sophisticated and informed methodology. In a worst-case scenario, a failure to recognise the fundamental differences between quantitative and qualitative approaches would result in a confused project with a muddled methodology and unclear research questions; conclusions about the research findings would be difficult to reach and possibly misleading. Other problems with combining qualitative and quantitative research in the same project include practical difficulties around collecting and analysing very different types of data and problems when structuring research reports. Mixed methods studies also tend to take a long time to complete and to be more costly in terms of needing expertise and infrastructure.

Debate continues about whether the two approaches can be successfully integrated in the same project or if instead they should be viewed as complementary but fundamentally separate approaches (Neuman 2000; Cresswell 2003). My advice, if you are considering combining qualitative and quantitative research, would be to consider your own level of expertise with qualitative and quantitative research (and those of other members of your research team, if working in a group). Qualitative research and quantitative research are both skilled activities, and as your skills grow and develop, your capacity to design and conduct complicated projects will also increase.

Above all, researchers should carefully weigh up the advantages and disadvantages of the various methods of social investigation and of mixed methods designs in relation to their research problem (Burgess 1993:106).

As with most other decisions about research, deciding if a mixed methods design is appropriate for your project and, if so, how it will be used is also a matter of personal taste, expectations arising from your discipline, and a reflection of your particular approach to research. These are all closely linked with the theoretical perspective(s) underpinning the project.

There are a number of commonly used ways to combine qualitative and quantitative research in health-related projects. These include using qualitative research as an exploratory stage in a larger quantitative project, using the two approaches to explore different aspects of the same research problem and comparing quantitative and qualitative research for the purpose of validation. Each of these techniques is explained in more detail below.

Exploratory stage

Qualitative research is well recognised as a useful first step in a larger quantitative project. The exploratory, inductive and interpersonal focus of qualitative research provides a useful way to learn about an unfamiliar setting or group of people (Pope & Mays 2000:3). Qualitative research can produce new ways of seeing an issue and may change the way a researcher views a problem (Morgan 1998). After conducting qualitative research, you may even find that a problem doesn't exist or that the problem you identified initially is far less important than a previously unrecognised one. The people-focused methods used in qualitative research mean that researchers can learn about the issue from the point of view of those intimately involved. This may include learning about language used by participants to talk about particular actions or behaviours (Hammersly 1990). Successful research projects where qualitative research has been used as an initial exploratory stage prior to the development of large questionnaires have shown the value of learning about how research participants use language before developing and administering a questionnaire (Jain et al. 2004; Wellings et al. 1994; Stone & Campbell 1986).

Investigating different aspects of the same problem

Pope and Mays (2000) and Sale et al. (2002) advocate using qualitative and quantitative research in a complementary way by investigating different aspects of the same research problem and by working in harmony to produce an additive outcome; that is, one impossible without the use of both approaches (Sale et al. 2002:50). A single project could incorporate several components as described above in the cigarette smoking example; some components make use of qualitative research, the others quantitative (Pope & Mays 2000:3). The results from these different methods may be discussed in relation to each other in order to produce new insights but are not used to confirm or validate each other. Instead they are recognised as offering alternative points of view and depth of understanding. 'Because the two paradigms do not study the same phenomena, quantitative and qualitative methods cannot be combined for cross-validation' (Sale et al. 2002:43).

This way of combining the two approaches has many benefits in areas of research such as nursing, primary care, public health, health education and health promotion where the complexity of issues means that no single approach is likely to produce sufficient insight (Baum 1995).

Validation

The third way that qualitative and quantitative research may be combined is when the results of qualitative research are used to 'validate' quantitative research. This design is strongly influenced by a positivist perspective. Combining the two approaches in this way can be seen as a form of triangulation (Mark & Shortland 1987). Begley (1996) recommends that mixed-method triangulation be used for cross-checking, confirming and validating findings and as a way of increasing the completeness of data. For example, the results from focus groups could be compared with results from a questionnaire to see if both types of research appear to be producing similar findings. The 'sequential use of qualitative and quantitative methods to develop and refine tools of enquiry may also be more effective for certain studies than the more usual simultaneous use' (Begley 1996:122). In a number of studies, results from qualitative research cast doubts on the validity of questionnaire data or, at the very least, prompt a reinterpretation of the questionnaire data (Jain et al. 2004; Pope & Mays 2003).

Nevertheless, comparing the results from two such different types of research for the purpose of validation is problematic to say the least. Because of the profound differences between quantitative and qualitative approaches, many qualitative researchers would question this use of mixed methods research (Sale et al. 2002; Sandelowski 1993).

> Triangulation relies on the notion of a fixed point, or superior explanation, against which other interpretations can be measured. Qualitative research, however, is usually carried out from a relativist perspective, which acknowledges the existence of multiple views of equal validity. Therefore, it does not readily lend itself to the production or observation of such a hierarchy of evidence. (Barbour 2001:1117)

Theory and qualitative research

As new researchers, one of the first things you are likely to notice about qualitative research is the explicit use of theory (Denzin & Lincoln 2003:3). Theories are sets of assumptions or related propositions that attempt to explain some domain of inquiry or phenomena. They are sometimes generalised and broad and can be applied to a wide range of situations, while others are specific and focused and designed only to address a limited range of situations (Grbich 1999:26–7). This difference is sometimes described as grand theory and theory of the middle range. Grand theory is abstract, comprehensive and widely applicable. Grand theories are large and often difficult to apply in qualitative research. Marxism and Structural Functionalism are both examples of grand theory. Theory of the middle range is less encompassing. It is suited to provide explanations or to guide inquiries about a specified phenomenon or situation. Most of the theory used by qualitative researchers to situate their work and provide a framework for analysis is middle range theory (Grbich 1999:27). Grbich also describes 'micro theory'. 'Micro theory consists of a set of hypothetical statements about a narrowly defined phenomenon. These statements are derived from interpretations of inter-related concepts' (1999:27). Micro theory is unlikely to be used when situating or interpreting qualitative research due to the narrowness of its scope. However, micro theory may be a product of research.

Qualitative researchers draw on theories from disciplines such as sociology, education, philosophy and anthropology. They also make use of theories developed specifically for qualitative research and they may develop their own theories based on their research.

> Qualitative inquirers use theory in their studies in several ways. They employ theory as a broad explanation, much like in quantitative research. This theory provides an explanation for behaviour and attitudes...

Alternatively, qualitative researchers increasingly use a theoretical lens or perspective to guide their study . . . They provide a lens (or even a theory) to guide the researchers as to what issues are important to examine . . . and the people that need to be studied . . . They also indicate how the researcher positions himself or herself in the qualitative study . . . and how the final written accounts need to be written. (Creswell 2003:131)

Qualitative research is characterised by theoretical plurality. In quantitative research, researchers use theory from a narrow range of disciplines, such as epidemiology, statistics and mathematics. While there is debate in these fields, this debate tends to be of interest to academics and theorists, while practitioners of research just get on and do their work. In contrast, consciously using theory from a wide range of disciplines and engaging in theoretical debate is integral to qualitative research (Denzin & Lincoln 1994). This is mainly *because* of the wide range of differing theoretical frameworks that underlie qualitative research. Even beginner researchers will find themselves reading and thinking theoretically, using ideas from sociological theory, feminist theory, philosophical theory and anthropological theory.

Theoretical plurality reflects and contributes to vigorous debate about the kinds of statements about the social world that can be made by qualitative researchers, what methods should be used to gain knowledge about the social world and what criteria this knowledge should meet (Blaikie 1993:6). It is usual for qualitative researchers to disagree about these issues to some extent. Different theoretical traditions are associated with different types of research questions, different types of data collection and analytic techniques and different styles of presentation of results. For qualitative researchers:

Theory is important. A theory provides a framework for explaining the way social forces work, for answering the question, 'Why?' Because we cannot study everything, the theory we choose determines what problems we will give priority to study, what direction we will consider most profitable to look for answers, and what kinds of data we will decide to collect. (McElroy & Townsend 1999:64)

Because different theoretical traditions make claims about what type of knowledge is desirable and how this knowledge can be best acquired, it is important that a researcher be aware of the theoretical underpinnings of the various methods they want to use (Rice & Ezzy 1999; Morse & Field 1996). Understanding alternative research paradigms will 'sensitise researchers and evaluators to the ways in which their methodological prejudices, derived from their disciplinary socialisation experiences, may reduce their methodological flexibility and adaptability' (Patton 1990:38). This issue is discussed in greater detail in Chapter Three.

Different research projects and different researchers make use of theory in different ways. How a researcher uses theory in any given research project is closely linked with the audience for the research and the motivations behind the research project.

Some projects are explicitly theoretically driven. This means that the researcher starts their project with the desire to make use of particular theory when investigating or exploring their chosen research problem or issue. This will impact on the decisions about research questions and, in turn, on the selection of appropriate methods. Consequently, assumptions about research underpinning the theoretical approach chosen by the researcher will make their choice of data collection and methods of analysis relatively straightforward.

Other research projects are largely method-driven. In such a project, the researcher knows from the outset that they want to make use of a particular qualitative method, often for pragmatic reasons (Brannen 1992:15). By selecting that method, they will be aligning themselves with theoretical approaches commonly associated with it and may need to refer to these in any written discussions outlining and justifying their methodology. Even projects where the researcher has made no explicit discussion of theory are still located within particular traditions; it may be that the researcher simply takes this position for granted as a 'normal' or 'desirable' way to conduct research (Rice & Ezzy 1999:11).

> This may not be a problem if there is an established research tradition in the field where such issues have been worked through. It may be that an established set of techniques has been used before to examine similar problems and the researcher only seeks similar sorts of answers. (Rice & Ezzy 1999:11)

Qualitative researchers often feel a commitment to a particular theoretical framework and conduct the majority of their research from within it. This is sometimes called a paradigm approach to qualitative research (Patton 1990:37–8; Lincoln & Guba 1985). If such an approach is considered legitimate in your discipline or research field, if it suits the purposes of your research and if it suits you, then this type of commitment can be highly productive, leading to a researcher becoming increasingly knowledgeable and expert. In contrast, other researchers prefer to adopt a pragmatic approach. They consider which theoretical position will be most appropriate for each particular research problem and then utilise qualitative methods and analytic techniques congruent with this approach. Patton describes this as 'methodological appropriateness' (1990:38). Researchers who adopt a pragmatic approach view various theoretical perspectives as 'instruments of analyses' (Foucault 1980:62 cited in Cheek 2000:2). However, some theoretical perspectives and their associated research methods and/or types of analysis do not sit easily together because they are so very different to each other. Because of this, researchers who adopt a pragmatic approach still need to be familiar with the most commonly used theoretical perspectives (Blaikie 1993:1).

The environment in which a researcher conducts their work also impacts on how they make use of theory. Research which is being conducted within an academic environment and where the results are to be published in certain peer-reviewed journals, books or as an academic thesis, generally makes much greater explicit use of theory than does applied research undertaken outside of academia. Academic research includes research conducted through universities and funded through government research bodies. These bodies review potential research projects using a panel of expert qualitative and quantitative researchers. The qualitative researchers on the panel will expect a researcher to demonstrate knowledge about the theories underpinning qualitative research and to locate their proposed research project within a pre-existing body of work and theory (Morse 1994; AHEC 1995).

In contrast, applied qualitative research conducted for lay audiences, such as the research conducted for health program evaluation, often makes little explicit use of theory. This is a reflection of the audience for this type of research, constraints on applied research in terms of available time and the skills of practitioners, and uncertainty about the usefulness of theory for the highly practical outcomes of much applied research (Brannen 1992; Shadish et al. 1991). Researchers involved in evaluation tend to be less interested in theory and more action-orientated than other researchers:

> If they rely on theories of evaluation at all in their work, it is to find prag-
> matic concepts to orientate them to their task and to suggest general
> strategies and some practical methods to implement those strategies. They
> want useful advice how to make their decisions given the constraints
> under which they work. (Shadish et al. 1991:57)

It must be emphasised, however, that while many applied researchers will conduct their work without making much reference to theory, they should, at a minimum, have knowledge of other research in their area of inquiry and be able to locate their work in relation to this (Rice & Ezzy 1999). The usual method of achieving this entails conducting a literature review, writing a discussion of it and incorporating this into a report of the research findings (*see* Chapter Two). Furthermore, evaluation is an increasingly sophisticated field of inquiry with an ever-growing body of disciplinary knowledge and associated theory related to qualitative research (such as Patton 1990; Patton 1997; Ovretveit 1998; Owen & Rogers 1999). As a result, expectations about the use of theory are changing. Theoretical perspectives often taken in evaluation or applied research to justify the use of certain qualitative research methods are fourth-generation evaluation (Guba & Lincoln 1989) and participatory action research (Kemmis & Wilkinson 1998).

As you can imagine, the need to understand and use theory poses considerable challenges for qualitative researchers without adequate training or familiarity with social science disciplines. Researchers working within these disciplines may also find the technical language obscure and the sheer volume of information available overwhelming. And the various books and articles about theory and qualitative research – all different from one another – are often confusing for new researchers. Authors frequently use the same term to refer to different phenomena or may vary in their interpretations and descriptions of various theoretical traditions. If you recognise that this is part and parcel of qualitative research, it may be easier to deal with the inevitable ambiguities associated with working in a research tradition marked by debate. I consider the variability within qualitative research a great strength – it provides opportunities for researchers to design innovative and challenging projects.

Chapter summary

This chapter provides background material essential for any new qualitative researcher. It describes research as a disciplined and systematic inquiry. It then introduces qualitative research as a distinct approach and describes the key differences between qualitative and quantitative research. Several of the issues and debates integral to qualitative research are introduced. Two major issues related to qualitative research are then discussed. The first of these is combining qualitative and quantitative research.

Mixed and multi-method research projects are common in health-related research. 'With the development and perceived legitimacy of both qualitative and quantitative research in the social and human sciences, mixed methods research, employing the data collection associated with both forms of data is expanding' (Creswell 2003:208). The challenges associated with designing and conducting mixed methods research are outlined and I emphasise the importance of clarity and careful planning in these types of complex study.

The second major issue discussed is the role of theory in qualitative research. Qualitative researchers use theory in a number of different ways. For example, theory is used to focus research and to raise research questions. Qualitative methodologies are often theory-driven, as is qualitative data analysis. The results from qualitative research may be expressed in terms of theory.

This chapter should prepare the reader for the following chapters and provoke an interest in qualitative research, leading to wider reading and discussion. The books appearing below in the list of recommended readings discuss the issues and topics presented in this chapter in greater detail.

Recommended reading

Cheek, J., Shoebridge, J., Willis, E. & Zadoroznyj, M. 1996, *Society and health: Social theory for health workers*, Longman Cheshire, Melbourne.

Denzin, N. & Lincoln, Y. 1994, *Handbook of qualitative research*, Sage Publications, Newbury Park, California.

Grbich, C. 1999, *Qualitative research in health: An introduction*, Allen & Unwin, Sydney.

Owen, J.M. & Rogers, P.K. 1999, *Program evaluation: Forms and approaches*, 2nd edn, Allen & Unwin, Sydney.

Patton, M.Q. 1990, *Qualitative evaluation and research methods*, 2nd edn, Sage Publications, Newbury Park, California.

Silverman, D. 1997, *Qualitative research: Theory, method and practice*, Sage Publications, London.

two

PLANNING YOUR RESEARCH

New researchers often find the thought of planning their research rather overwhelming. I must admit it does tend to be a complex and time-consuming process. However, the benefits of carefully planning a research project will be evident in the quality of the results (Ward & Holman 2001). As with most complex tasks, it is easier to plan a research project if it is broken down into smaller sections. Luckily, the majority of health-related qualitative research projects follow a predictable research process with a number of distinct stages. These stages are common across a wide range of differing methodologies, subject areas and types of research project. They are identifying a research problem and initial questions; conducting a literature review; clarifying research questions; developing a research plan; reflecting on ethics and adapting the plan in response to feedback from an ethics review committee; acquiring funding; data collection and analysis; and disseminating research findings.

In this chapter each of these stages will be described in detail with suggestions about key issues for a beginning researcher to consider as they work on their own projects. The chapter concludes with a case study from Lisa Crossland. Lisa is a primary healthcare researcher from a regional university. Her case study demonstrates the way that she used qualitative research in the evaluation of an after-hours primary care service.

The research process

It is helpful to think of research in terms of a process that can be broken down into distinct stages. Some of these stages may occur concurrently while others cannot occur until previous stages have been completed. In the majority of projects, there are at least four important stages to complete before any data is collected.

Stage 1
Identify a research problem or field of inquiry – and possibly some preliminary research questions.
Stage 2
Conduct a literature review and refine your research questions.
Stage 3
Develop and write a plan for your research, outlining methodology, methods, ethical issues and any required infrastructure.
Stage 4
Obtain ethical clearance from an ethics committee or institutional review board, if needed. Otherwise, at a minimum, with a reference group, advisory group or supervisor, discuss ethical issues and how these will be overcome.
Stage 5
Apply for funding, if necessary. Most applications for competitive funding require a research plan and ethical clearance.
Stage 6
Undertake data collection and analysis, and document research processes and findings. Obviously, this is the largest stage in a research project. In many qualitative projects, collection and analysis occur concurrently.
Stage 7
Disseminate your research findings.

Identifying a research problem

Identifying a research problem is the first stage in the research process. In some research situations, researchers are given a pre-existing problem and asked to design a project to address it. This often happens to applied researchers conducting an evaluation or in projects where researchers are building on earlier work. At other times, researchers find themselves in the daunting position of being told to find something interesting and important and then to research it. This investigator-driven situation is often associated with research undertaken for the purpose of academic study, such as a research higher degree. Such open-ended choice strikes me as difficult, as the number of issues that I find fascinating seems to be infinite!

Either way, a research problem should be something that absorbs you. A personal interest will help carry you through the difficult times and the inevitable crises or dull times. It should also be of interest to a wider audience because research (as discussed in Chapter One) is part of a larger process of finding answers and generating new knowledge (Pryke et al. 2003; Whitworth 1994). The size and nature of this audience will vary widely depending on the type of research you are planning to undertake. For example, it could range from a group of your colleagues and other researchers in your institution or workplace to a funding body, members of your academic discipline or even governments (i.e. national priority areas for research). Research problems are often quite broad; for example, 'identifying reasons for falls in the elderly', 'lowering the rates of childhood obesity', 'improving the health of disadvantaged children' or 'preventing teenage smoking'.

A research problem defines the area of inquiry and hopefully sets parameters about what the research project is aiming to achieve (Creswell 2003). It may also lead to some preliminary research questions. However, these will require further development and clarification. Where a research problem indicates a field of inquiry, research questions indicate how the research will actually be done. Research questions are more detailed and focused than research problems because they need to be answerable through the research project and are linked to data collection methods. This means that developing research questions will involve consideration about the type of research you want to conduct (e.g. methods used and study population).

Initially, you will probably quickly develop one or more rough research questions. This can be a useful way to get started, and the questions might call to mind certain peers or experts with whom it would be helpful to talk about the research. I cannot overemphasise the importance of collaboration at this early stage. Research is not a solitary occupation, and the advice of others is invaluable, as I know from experience. For example, when I started my current research position, I quickly learnt that speaking with medical doctors about the practicality of conducting research in general practice and hospital settings made a huge difference when designing 'achievable' projects (Hansen 2001; Hansen & Robinson 2003; Hansen et al. 2004). As a novice researcher, you are likely to have some degree of research guidance 'on tap'. This could be an academic supervisor, a reference group or your colleagues. Make use of them. Discussing your work with others will be to your benefit – as they ask you to elaborate and explain, you will be forced to decide exactly what you *really* want to know about your chosen research problem.

Literature review

Conducting a literature review will help you to find out what other work has been done on your research problem or similar problems (Ward & Holman 2001). Doing a literature review entails researching your topic in academic journals, monographs, conference proceedings and textbooks. When you speak with colleagues about your research, they will probably suggest useful books or journals. You may also have a small library of your own. These can be useful places to start. However, the quickest and most efficient way to search the literature is to visit a good library and use its catalogues and on-line databases. These will enable you to search for topics, authors and keywords across a wide range of sources. Library catalogues are used to locate journals and textbooks held by your library. Many journals are also available in electronic forms, and full-text versions of articles can be downloaded. On-line databases are used to identify suitable articles, journals and books wherever they are held. Examples of these databases include PubMed, Sociological Abstracts, Web of Science and CINHAL. Most databases only go back about 15 years, and some do not cover textbooks and monographs. Be aware of this when conducting a literature review and if you need to use non-academic texts or locate the results from older research, consider using additional library catalogues and the reference lists from older books or articles.

In some instances, it can also be valuable to read theses and govern-ment/non-government reports. These are rarely found in health-related on-line databases and may not be listed in library catalogues. Websites for government agencies often include publication lists for reports and government publications. It may also be necessary to write to a specific agency or organisation requesting copies of reports. If unsure about searching or locating any literature sources, ask a librarian for help. They are specially trained in this issue and in many libraries they offer training sessions (Creswell 2003:38).

After you have identified the key literature, you need to take the time to actually read some of it and to skim over other parts. Initially, you should search, read and skim to find out what questions other researchers have asked and how they investigated them. You may find that the answers you seek are already out there. This doesn't mean that you will need to abandon your research project but it may provide an opportunity to change your focus slightly.

Of course, you may find that no research has been done on your research problem. Sometimes it is difficult to interpret the meaning of this. Does it mean that no-one else has recognised the problem? Or is it a reflection of current trends in the field? Has something changed in the social or political climate around you, pushing that particular research problem to your attention at this point in time? Perhaps your problem is not of interest to others? It's worth considering these issues as they will all impact on your ability to publish your research findings and attract research funding. Either way, a lack of existing research into your chosen research problem suggests an opportunity.

Reading about research done by other researchers is also one of the best ways to find out what research methods are considered credible and legitimate in your field (Merriam 1998). For example, in some health-related fields, qualitative research is rarely conducted. If you discover that no-one from your field has addressed your research problem using qualitative methods, it can feel quite exciting, but it is also a warning signal that you may need to be fairly conservative in your approach, or combine qualitative with quantitative methods if you hope to obtain competitive grant money or to publish results in certain journals (Morse 1994). Conversely, if your problem has been widely researched by qualitative researchers, you may need to develop an innovative approach to make your research of interest to others.

Reviewing the literature can also give you a lot of new ideas for your research. For example, after reading around your topic, you may realise that the way you were considering the problem has changed or you may have learnt about a new research method you hadn't been aware of before. For this reason, it is important that you conduct a literature review that is not limited to your own particular academic discipline, such as medicine or nursing. Other fields, such as sociology, psychology, allied health, geography or education, will contain studies that may be extremely useful for your research project (Merriam 1998).

If you are doing an honours degree, a research higher degree or preparing a report from your research, you will be expected to write a formal and comprehensive literature review. This has several objectives. First, it is an overview of existing research. Second, it should present an argument about why your research is important or necessary. Third, it should include a review of literature focused on qualitative research and a discussion about your methodology (Locke et al. 2000).

If you are presenting your research findings in the form of a published article or conference paper, you will be expected to briefly review the literature. As this will have to be fully up-to-date, keep in mind the need to search for new literature regularly over the course of your research project. I have often found that when a problem suddenly seems impor-tant and interesting to me, it will have caught the attention of other researchers in my field at the same time. This can result in a plethora of publications about a single issue occurring at roughly the same time.

Clarifying research questions

After doing some reading and talking to others, you should be much closer to deciding exactly what it is you want to know and writing it down in the form of research questions. These should be expressed as clearly as possible (Ward & Holman 2001:60). Avoid double-barrelled questions.

Clarifying research questions is an important stage in a qualitative research project for several reasons. A research question narrows the focus of a broadly stated research problem and consequently guides the project. This is the stage in the research process where a researcher decides who the participants for the study should be and what data collection methods are the most suitable (Creswell 2003:204–5). Furthermore, research questions are equivalent to the formal hypotheses or research objectives used in quantitative research.

Cresswell (2003:104–8) makes a number of important recommendations about developing qualitative research questions. He suggests that researchers avoid starting a question with the word 'why', instead choosing emergent and open terms such as 'what' or 'how'. He also recommends that researchers choose terms that reflect a qualitative methodology. For example, 'describe', 'discover', 'understand' and 'explore' are preferable to words that suggest a quantitative study, such as 'influence', 'impact', 'determine', 'cause' and 'relate'. Research questions in qualitative studies are often expressed using a central or core research question(s) followed by a number of sub-questions that may relate explicitly to different research methods. For the purpose of guiding a research project, a core research question does not have to be expressed in the form of a question. It is possible to use a clearly defined problem statement instead. For example:

Core questions
- Do women and general practitioners share similar understandings about the implications of abnormal pap smear results?
- How do female teenage smokers describe 'taking up' smoking cigarettes?

Core purpose statements
- To describe the experience of being diagnosed with breast cancer.
- To explore the relationship between being a parent and living with a chronic disease.
- The intent of this project is to better understand parental decision making about childhood immunisation.

Core questions should be followed with a number of more closely focused statements or questions that specify what you want to know plus what type of data you plan to collect. For example:

- How do women who have received abnormal pap smear results in the previous 12 months describe the meanings of these results and their perceptions of cervical cancer risk during a semi-structured interview?
- How do general practitioners describe the meanings of various abnormal smear results shown to them during a semi-structured interview?
- How do they talk about cervical cancer risk during the interview?
- What understandings related to pap smear results and cervical cancer risk are apparent in focus groups with women who have received an abnormal pap smear result in the previous 12 months?
- What understandings related to pap smear results and cervical cancer risk are apparent in focus groups with general practitioners?

As you can see, developing research questions requires knowledge about research methods and methodology. These topics are explained in detail in the following chapters.

Research plan

The next stage of the research process is the development of a research plan. The research problem, questions, methodology and methods are pulled together into a research plan. All research projects need a research plan (also called a research proposal, or protocol). The act of writing even a short plan is a necessary stage in the research process because it helps a researcher to clarify what they are researching and how they will go about it (Lock et al. 2000; Punch 1998). Research plans are also required for a number of pragmatic reasons. Any research project conducted for a graduate or postgraduate degree has to have a written plan, which is assessed or used to decide who gains entry to the course. Furthermore, most qualitative research projects require some type of formal ethical approval before any data can be collected (Rice & Ezzy 1999; Punch 1998). The ethical approval process involves submitting a research plan to an ethics committee. Obtaining competitive research funding always requires a written research plan. In the applied arena, an evaluation also requires a plan, and this may form part of a competitive tender, be integrated into the original program plan or submitted to a reference or advisory group (Ovretveit 1998).

Below are annotated outlines for two research plans. The first is well suited to any type of academic qualitative research. This includes projects for which competitive funding and publication in peer-reviewed journals is sought. The second is more appropriate to a qualitative evaluation. Researchers can tailor both of these outlines to suit their project. Creswell (2003) and Lock et al. (2000) both contain detailed discussions about developing research plans. Remember that when planning a qualitative research project, changes in the research design may occur during the course of the project. Because of this you may find yourself having to change and adapt your plan as the research is conducted. In the case of an ongoing evaluation, changing client needs may mean that several new plans are developed over time.

Academic qualitative research plan

A title

This should be descriptive and may change by the end of the research project.

Significant statement

State the research problem and briefly say why it is important or significant. This should be no more than one or two paragraphs.

Research questions

The type of qualitative study you plan to conduct will influence the level of detail. For example, a highly inductive grounded theory study would have exploratory and possibly quite generalised questions, while a focused observation study would have more specific and detailed questions.

Literature review

In some proposals, this section might not be necessary and could be replaced entirely by the significance statement. In others, a more detailed literature review is required. Remember to include a full reference list at the end of the plan.

Methodology

This section should justify and explain the choice of methods and describe how the research questions were developed. This will involve describing the disciplinary background to the methods and approaches chosen and detailing their use in other similar studies (Creswell 2003:183; Morse 1994). Also discuss any potential ethical issues and how these will be dealt with. Some plans will require a separate section on ethics. It is important to outline the researcher's role in the study. In some studies, this may also necessitate a discussion about the researcher's own attitudes, experiences and personal beliefs relating to the study.

Data collection methods

Clearly describe methods of data collection and give details about the research participants, the site or locations at which the research will be conducted, plus any relevant information about how the participants/sites were selected for the study and how data will be recorded. Explain how the methods will address the research questions. You will also need to include information about how participants will be contacted and any strategies in place for gaining access to the field (see following chapters for details on these).

Data analysis

Clearly describe the proposed methods of analysis and interpretation. Creswell (2003:191–2) recommends that qualitative analysis be broken down into generic steps when writing a research plan. These might include organising and preparing the data, an exploratory reading stage and then any specific analytic techniques, such as coding, searching for narratives or using a particular software program (2003:192). Spend some time detailing any strategies used to increase reliability and validity, if this suits your project; for example, member checks or triangulation of data (*see* Chapter Three).

Expected outcomes

This section may include reference to concrete outcomes, such as designing a questionnaire or change in practice arising from a partici-patory action research project, or less concrete outcomes, such as increased disciplinary knowledge about a particular problem or issue or providing a basis for larger studies in the future. Mention any possible applied uses for the research and discuss any plans to publish from the research.

Appendices

These may include copies of draft interview guides, focus group questions, observation schedules, maps etc. Also a timeline and budget. These are not necessary for all projects. The budget might include the cost of any recording equipment, travel or transcription if the researcher does not plan on doing this themselves.

Plan for a qualitative evaluation

The following plan is suitable for an evaluation. It is adapted from Ovretveit (1998:66–72). This plan would also be suited to some types of applied qualitative research projects as it tends to be focused around pragmatic issues, such as budget, audience and concrete outcomes.

Specifying the evaluand

This section should outline the focus of the evaluation and explain why the evaluation is being done.

Audience for the evaluation

Describing the primary audience for the evaluation. 'The primary audience is the individual or group that is most likely to use the knowledge, in the form of findings, conclusions or recommendations' (1998:68). It is important to specify this clearly.

Resources, budget and timelines

This is an important section in the plan for an evaluation project. Ovretveit (1998:70) suggests that a week-by-week schedule that includes likely costs is a useful approach.

Evaluation focus

This section could describe what elements of the program will be evaluated and why. It may also include a short literature review outlining findings and methods from other similar evaluations or programs.

Evaluation questions and methods

Clearly outline the key questions and describe the methods that will be used to address each of these. Avoid the temptation to skim over details related to methodology. In particular, it is important that you address the type of qualitative research strategy to be used and provide some background information about the history of the approach, and that you address appropriateness and the strengths and weaknesses of the approach for this evaluation.

Detailed data management

This section is akin to the methods sections in the academic research plan above. It should describe the methods in detail and explain why they are appropriate. This section could also cover issues such as codes of behaviour and ethics, and sampling (if appropriate), and describe clearly how the data will be analysed in order to address the evaluation questions (Ovretveit 1998:72). As with the plan above, I advise breaking the analysis process into generic steps that will be understandable, even to those without knowledge of qualitative analysis.

Describing how results will be disseminated

This section of a plan entails specifying how the evaluation results will be disseminated and who will do this. Ovretveit suggests that innovative and thoughtful dissemination strategies are important if evaluations are to have an impact on decision making. He considers that long reports have only a limited utility and other methods that 'allow clients and evaluators to interact' are more successful (1998:70).

Ethics

The ethical considerations associated with research are largely aimed at protecting research participants from any harm associated with their involvement in the research. However, conducting ethical research also requires researcher integrity and a commitment to basic ethical principles such as a respect for persons, beneficence and justice. The rigour and suitability of the methods used are also ethical issues (Neuman 1994:427). For example, an ethical researcher will avoid collecting unnecessary information about research participants, misusing research results or using biased recruitment related to issues such as sexual orientation, race, ethnicity, gender or disability.

Ethics and ethical principles extend to all spheres of human activity. They should apply to our dealings with each other, with animals and the environment. They should govern our interactions not only in conducting research but also in commerce, employment and politics. Ethics serve to identify good, desirable or acceptable conduct and provide reasons for those conclusions. (National Health and Medical Research Council 1999:1)

The same 'ethical principles apply to all forms of research involving humans' (National Health and Medical Research Council 1995:3). In recognition of the importance of ethics to research, organisations such as universities, government departments, hospitals and some professional associations have ethics committees (also called institutional review boards). The purpose of these groups is to review research plans and identify any ethically problematic aspects of the research (Loff & Black 2004). They also make suggestions about how these problematic aspects can be overcome. Formal approval from an ethics committee is desirable for all research projects. Approval from an ethics committee is essential for researchers undertaking a degree or research higher degree, when applying for competitive grant funding and when the researcher wants results from the project to be published in peer-refereed journals or presented at reputable conferences. For these reasons, gaining ethical clearance is a necessary step for almost all research projects.

Research-related organisations and professional bodies have statements and guidelines for those involved in conducting research. Guidelines for conducting ethical qualitative research can also be accessed using qualitative research websites and in textbooks such as Denzin and Lincoln 1994, Grbich 1999 and Punch 1998. Many countries have a set of national guidelines outlining ethical principles and procedures. In Australia, for instance, these are provided by the National Health and Medical Research Council (NHMRC).

Guidelines or statements are especially helpful when preparing applications to be presented to an ethics committee. For some projects, the application of specified ethical guidelines may be mandatory. Your research supervisors will also assist you to recognise and address any ethical issues associated with your project.

If you are conducting your research outside of an institution with its own ethics committee, you may still be able to make use of an ethics committee associated with your profession (such as nursing, general practice, public health or epidemiology), a teaching hospital or a university. Some government departments also have ethics committees that may agree to review your work. If you are conducting research outside the auspices of any ethics committee or without direct supervision from a more experienced researcher, you still have a responsibility to inform yourself about the ethical and legal aspects of qualitative research. Keep in mind that research conducted outside the auspices of an ethics committee or institutional review board may be impossible to publish in academic journals or to present at academic conferences.

Several key ethical issues associated with qualitative research are briefly outlined below (Richards & Schwartz 2002; Cutliffe & Ramcharan 2002).

Informed consent

It is important that, before giving their consent to participate in research, participants fully understand what their involvement will entail, the purpose of the study and what will happen to their private information. They should also be aware of their right to request that their data be excluded from the study. The usual informed consent model includes several steps (Marvasti 2004:139):

1 Potential participant provided with an information sheet about the study, outlining possible risks, explaining what will happen with data, details about confidentiality.
2 If they agree to participate, they and the investigator sign a consent form.
3 Participation is voluntary, without coercion or inducement.
4 Withdrawal from the study is possible at any time without ill effect.

The information sheet provided to potential research participants consists of a general description of the project, a list of identified potential harms and benefits, and an explanation about how their confidentiality or anonymity will be protected. This information sheet should also emphasise that participation in the research is voluntary and withdrawal is possible at any stage without penalty. If the potential participant decides to become an actual participant, they are asked to sign a consent form. These forms and the information sheets generally follow standard templates and have to be approved by an ethics committee or institutional review board.

Another key aspect of the informed consent model is the understanding that participants should not be subject to any 'coercion, or to any inducement or influence' which could impair their voluntary character (NHMRC 1999:12). This aspect of informed consent is designed to prevent unethical situations such as restricting access to medical care if people do not agree to participate in research or paying participants large sums of money if they agree to undergo potentially dangerous tests or to trial new medications. The issue of inducement is extremely complex. In projects, certain researchers or research participants may want to include some form of compensation or payment for participants. Paying those who participate in research can be coercive, particularly if they are poor or in need of money. However, not recognising the value of a participant's research input or the costs associated with their participation in the research (e.g. time away from work or travel costs) may be insulting and create difficulties for recruitment. Ethics committees often have clear guidelines on this issue, and researchers will need to follow these. In addition, researchers need to consider this issue for themselves and justify their decisions about payment or compensation based on the needs and characteristics of people involved in their research. For instance, it may be reasonable to compensate parents for the cost of childcare for the time that the parents are travelling to, attending and returning from a focus group.

The informed consent model was developed to meet the needs of quantitative and medical research. It is a valuable process; however, there are difficulties in applying some aspects of it in qualitative research projects. These largely arise because of the flexible and slightly unpredictable nature of qualitative research. For example, it is difficult to specify interview questions or the nature of focus group interaction ahead of time. The signed consent model is also more difficult to apply in ethnographic research where a researcher might have a number of informal interviews or interactions with people who have not read an information sheet or even provided the researcher with their names. Most qualitative researchers find that obtaining consent is a continuous process during a research project. In projects where data collection continues over time and the situations of the participants may be changing, researchers should not automatically assume that each individual's consent is ongoing (Lawton 2001).

Right to privacy/confidentiality

This is a normal requirement for the majority of social research, whether it is quantitative or qualitative. Confidentiality can be understood as 'the obligation of persons to whom private information has been given not to use the information for any purpose other than that for which it was given' (NHMRC 1999:62). It also refers to participant anonymity; that is, that research participants cannot be identified in research results. This is often achieved by using pseudonyms for people and places. Demographic tables listing participants (or pseudonyms) and variables such as age, number of children, gender etc should be used with great care as those familiar with the study may be able to identify participants using this information. Qualitative studies require particularly complex strategies to ensure anonymity and confidentiality. Strategies include combining responses from different participants to form a composite or excluding certain pieces of data from the study because anonymity cannot be guaranteed.

> Of course, it is understood that anonymity, like secrecy, is a matter of degree. In intensive interview studies, public place observations, or studies of fluid social groupings, individuals may be able to identify quotations from or descriptions of themselves. They are extremely unlikely to be able to identify anyone else. In studies of stable communities or ongoing groups however, pseudonyms are unlikely to prevent any of the participants from recognising or at least making pretty accurate guesses about 'who's who'. (Lofland & Lofland 1984:29)

Qualitative data collection methods, like interviews, focus groups and participant observation, pose challenges for researchers in terms of confidentiality and privacy (Cutcliffe & Ramcharan 2002). Qualitative methods are often interactive, so researchers rarely work with anonymous data. The identities of research participants are usually known to the researchers and frequently also to the people transcribing the data (Richards & Schwartz 2002). Relationships formed between researchers and research participants are likely to be complex and may continue in some form after the project is finished. The line between information obtained as research data and information arising from friendship or being an acquaintance is likely to be unclear at least some of the time in ethnographic studies or other studies involving ongoing contact. In addition, research participants may find it difficult to maintain the confidentiality of other participants. For example, focus group participants do not always maintain the confidentiality of other participants, despite agreeing to do so during the focus group.

Protection from harm

Harm arising from poorly conducted research can range from physical injury and emotional distress to the risk of scandal or libel suits associated with disclosing information about issues such as sexuality, behaviour or illegal activity. The type of harm most often discussed in relation to qualitative research is the potential for qualitative projects to cause emotional distress to participants (Corbin & Morse 2003). However, this risk can usually be overcome by sensitive and thoughtful researchers and, if needed, by arranging counselling for participants (Rice & Ezzy 1999:39). Study participants may find their participation to be a positive and beneficial experience because of, or despite, the sensitive nature of the research. Scott et al. (2002) invited 97 people who had previously participated in an interview-based study focused on the experience of having a child diagnosed with Ewing's sarcoma to complete a self-administered questionnaire designed to investigate how participation in the former study had affected them. Eighty-one people completed the questionnaire. Almost all stated they were glad they had participated in the research as it had given them 'the opportunity to discuss their child's illness and that the knowledge gained' because of their participation 'would benefit others' (2002:509).

Researchers need to take time to consider any negative repercussions for participants (in addition to emotional distress) that may arise as a consequence of their participation. Research has great potential to be exploitative (Marvasti 2004). Qualitative research, because of inter-personal contact and the potentially intimate nature of the knowledge shared, is particularly vulnerable to this. Sometimes the consequences of participating in research can be far-reaching, impacting on the researcher and the research participants in unexpected ways (Warren 1977; Marvasti 2004:134–5).

Covert fieldwork

If you read about qualitative research conducted during the 1950s and 1960s, you will find many fascinating examples of research where the researcher went 'under cover' in some way while conducting their research; for example, Goffman (1961). However, since the 1970s any type of deliberate deception has generally been considered potentially unethical research conduct. Clear conflicts exist between expectations about informed consent and any covert or 'secretive' social research; for example, when a researcher joins a group in order to conduct observation and informal interviewing for a research project without informing members of the organisation about this purpose. So how do qualitative researchers resolve this issue? Well, first, covert fieldwork has largely gone 'out of fashion'. Expectations that any research involving humans requires informed consent makes it extremely difficult to ever gain approval from an ethics committee for any types of deliberate deception.

Second, a largely informal rule exists whereby covert qualitative research can be conducted using publicly available documents and using observation/participant observation in public/open spaces, such as sporting events and bus stops, without the need for informed consent.

However, ethical problems are seen to arise when the research involves talking with people, collecting personal information and in any shifts 'out of the public realm and into the private' (Lofland & Lofland 1984:22). Covert fieldwork remains a contested issue:

> Our view is that there are very serious, perhaps damning, ethical problems in all covert research if the presumed immorality of deception is the overriding concern. Deception is no less present in public and open settings than in preplanned 'deep cover' research in closed settings. On the other hand, if other concerns are also important (for example, lack of harm to those researched or the theoretical importance of a setting that can never be studied openly), then we find no more justification for abolishing all deep cover research, than for abolishing secret research in public settings. (Lofland & Lofland 1984:23)

A general rule of thumb for beginning researchers is to avoid any type of covert fieldwork. However, if you have a project that may involve some degree of covertness, I recommend discussing the issue with your research supervisors and reading both Punch (1986) and Diener and Crandall (1978) to help you decide if the covertness can be justified. You will also need to be closely guided by an ethics committee.

Vulnerable participants

Certain people are considered to be particularly vulnerable to exploitation and other types of harm or risk associated with their participation in research. These include children, older people, indigenous people, those in dependent or unequal relationships, people highly dependent on medical care, pregnant women, people living in poverty and those with an intellectual disability or impaired capacity to communicate (Grbich 1999:74–6). The special needs of these population groups should be considered and the research designed appropriately (Marvasti 2004).

Other issues

In addition to the topics listed above, many other ethical issues may arise during the course of a qualitative research project that may not be covered in formal ethical applications but that are nonetheless important (Sieber 1998; Lofland & Lofland 1984).

> As qualitative researchers often have indepth interactions with participants over a long period of time, the nature of the researcher–participant

relationship needs special consideration. Specifically, a close researcher–participant relationship evokes concerns about perceived coercion, experiences of undue burden or distress, and privacy issues. (NIH 2005:12)

In my experience, the best way to approach unclear ethical issues is to think more about your research participants and less about your own wants or needs. In addition, before you start your research it is worth spending some time thinking about how you see your role as a researcher and how you think research should be conducted. For example, how willing are you to get involved with your research participants? What do you regard to be manipulation? What behaviours would you consider to be unsuitable for a researcher or a research participant? How will you deal with any difficult or unexpected situations that may arise?

Grbich (1999:101) suggests that before a researcher starts collecting data, they should also put time into planning how they might deal with unpleasant or uncomfortable situations, such as embarrassment, racism or sexual harassment. It is also possible that as a researcher you will have to make judgments about what to do with information acquired as a consequence of the research. Researchers carry a legal obligation to report to authorities information about child abuse, violence or unlawful activity. The specifics of these will vary across jurisdictions. It may be that your research reveals levels of neglect, abuse or malpractice that are not sufficient to clearly invite formal legal action. What should you do then? Such questions have particular relevance for healthcare practitioners.

> For health care practitioners, confidentiality means that no personal information is passed on except in exceptional circumstances. For researchers, the extent of the duty of confidentiality is less clear (though often assumed to be absolute), and this difference can lead to conflict for practitioner/researchers. (Richards & Schwartz 2002)

Practitioners are also likely to experience ethically ambiguous situations when conflicts arise between their role as a provider of healthcare and their role as a researcher. For example, research participants involved in a project focused around a disease or condition frequently ask researchers for advice about medication, treatment or healthcare providers. How should you respond if you do, in fact, have the information they are requesting? Conducting research in medical settings where you also work as a healthcare professional may place you in an overly powerful position in relation to the research participants. Your role as a healthcare professional and an expert person who works in that setting might eclipse your role as researcher. And if, as a health professional, you consider that a research participant is too unwell to continue being interviewed or involved in a participant observation but they state they want to continue, what would you do?

Strategies to deal with these types of event include brainstorming with colleagues, being fully informed about legal responsibilities and having up-to-date information about services and support groups. It may also be helpful to take heed of the following advice given by Davies and Dodd (2002):

> Understanding ethics to involve trustfulness, openness, honesty, respect-fulness, carefulness, and constant attentiveness means ethics is not treated as a separate part of our research – a form that is filled in for ethics committees and forgotten . . . an implicit part of ethical practice thus involves the acknowledgment and location of the researcher within the research process. (Davies & Dodd 2002:281)

Funding

Not all researchers have to apply for funding; perhaps the project they are working on is small, with no need for a large budget, or it may be already funded. This might apply to students, to researchers who have been contracted to conduct research for others, or to people conducting small evaluations or research projects within their own organisation. However, after developing a research plan and either gaining ethical clearance or at least arranging to do so, many researchers will need to obtain funding for their research (Morse 1994: 220–35). For instance, professional and university-based researchers often apply for competitive research grants from various grant and institutional bodies, health-related organisations and industry partners, such as pharmaceutical companies. Postgraduate students often have to apply for competitive scholarship funding. Healthcare providers may need to apply for funding to pay for large evaluations.

There are a number of ways that a qualitative researcher can increase their chances of obtaining funding (Morse 1994: 220–35). It is vital to find out the criteria used to review applications in the funding round you have chosen and to tailor your application appropriately. It can also be useful to learn the history of the grant and to establish the motivations of the people or group providing the funding. This may lead to a shift in the emphasis of your project or it could be helpful when selecting research problems to investigate. If you are applying for competitive research funding (not a scholarship), you will need to build a research team with a proven track record in the area and type of research that you propose to investigate. Above all, qualitative research proposals must be clearly expressed and rigorous. A common criticism of qualitative research applications submitted to funding rounds is that they lack clarity or that methods or analysis are poorly explained. Others tips include:

- Allow plenty of time to complete your application.
- Ask for advice; if possible, look at other successful applications.
- Acknowledge the limitations of your research but stress the benefits of your approach.
- Avoid the use of jargon.
- Be aware that you may need to apply to more than one agency, apply more than once or fund different aspects of the research at various times.

Data collection and analysis

Finally, after all the reading, planning and discussion, a researcher arrives at the stage in the research process where they start collecting and analysing data. Detailed accounts of qualitative data collection and data analysis methods are provided in later chapters of this book. A number of predictable tasks are involved with the data collection and data analysis stage.

Selecting and recruiting research participants and gaining access to the research site

Before any data can be collected, researchers have to contact research participants and gain permission to access any locations, documents or groups of people involved with the research. While decisions about sampling and contact methods were made during the research planning process, actually finding research participants and getting them to participate is rarely straightforward. As Lofland and Lofland (1984:20) describe it, 'when decision is translated into action, when your intention to do research is translated into beginning that research, then you encounter the first truly *social* moment of naturalistic investigation: getting in – gaining acceptance of the people being studied'.

Collecting and recording data

A qualitative research project is likely to use one or more of the following data collection methods – interviewing, observation, focus groups, documents and mixed qualitative/quantitative. Each of these will require considerable personal effort (in terms of time, planning and social interaction) by the researcher.

Then data needs to be recorded in some way so that the researcher can review it later and so that their research findings are accountable and transparent. Recording data might involve a combination of audio recording then transcription; video recording or photographing; observation schedules; journals; and field notes. Data recording is incredibly important in qualitative research. A systematic and rigorous approach to data recording is one of the characteristics that differentiate research from normal interaction and armchair theorising about the social world (Lofland & Lofland 1984).

Managing and keeping track of data

As data is collected and recorded, it is a responsibility of the researcher to maintain it and keep track of it. Data management includes recording data in an appropriate format for the methods of analysis chosen, labelling and sorting data sets, keeping data safe, and fulfilling requirements about confidentiality and data security. There are many different tools that can be used to assist with these tasks. These include filing systems, index cards, databases and purpose-built computer software programs designed for managing and analysing qualitative data (*see* Chapter Seven). Well-organised data greatly assists with data analysis. It is also important to maintain records in a safe and confidential manner. Many institutions require research data to be kept for up to ten years after the completion of the research (Sieber 1998).

Analysing and interpreting data

In iterative qualitative research projects, data collection and analysis occur in tandem. However, in most projects the completion of data collection signals the beginning of a phase of the research when the researcher can focus their energies on analysis. There are many recognised methods and approaches used in qualitative research to guide the analysis and interpretation of data (*see* Chapter Seven). Among these are iterative thematic analysis, content analysis, narrative analysis and discourse analysis. While the researcher will have made decisions about these as they designed the methodology and research plan for their project, given the flexibile nature of qualitative research, it is likely that a researcher's original plans for data analysis will be adapted or changed over the duration of the research. As with data management, analysis may involve the use of a computer program (Coffey & Atkinson 1996; Taft 1993).

Disseminating research findings

Dissemination is the process by which knowledge arising from research is transmitted to appropriate target audiences. These audiences may include other researchers, healthcare practitioners, policy makers, the public, regulatory bodies and funding bodies. Ideally, consideration about the dissemination of research will occur during the early planning stages of a research project. Some grants and funding bodies expect researchers to think strategically and politically about dissemination and research uptake. They will take this into consideration when ranking applications (Morse & Field 1996:141).

Frequently used methods of disseminating research results are peer-reviewed journals, conference presentations, reports, theses, newsletters, oral presentations, websites, guidelines, emails, academic detailing and mailed handouts. Researchers tend to stick with simple dissemination strategies or neglect dissemination altogether. This is unfortunate because dissemination is a vital stage in the research process (King et al. 1996). As stated in Chapter One, research does not exist in isolation. The results of research (including information about how methods were used) need to be available for scrutiny and to make a contribution to wider stocks of knowledge.

> In many ways, the ultimate impact of your planned project rests in the effectiveness of your dissemination strategy . . . The underlying reason to gain and then disseminate new research-based information is to assure it is appropriately considered for use in making decisions, making changes, or taking other specific actions designed to improve outcomes. That is, the goal of dissemination is *utilisation*. (National Institute on Disability and Rehabilitation Research 2001:4)

When planning how to disseminate your research, the task is identifying the goals and objectives for your dissemination effort. You may find that you have a number of these. They could include gaining a peer-reviewed publication for your curriculum vitae, informing other researchers in your field, meeting reporting requirements associated with funding and providing feedback for research participants and colleagues. After identifying these goals, you will need to decide exactly what information you want to convey to each audience and the best ways of doing this. Different audiences often require different methods of dissemination (Richardson 2003; Rice & Ezzy 1999). For example, it is unlikely that consumers will read academic peer-reviewed journals, and policy makers won't be able to use your research if it was only distributed in an internal report within your organisation.

Bear in mind the following when thinking about disseminating your research. Always try to match your target audiences with the appropriate medium or media. Never underestimate the value of talking with people about your research. In many instances, this is a particularly effective means of dissemination. The users of your research findings are more likely to take in information and ideas from sources they perceive as credible and trustworthy. Effective dissemination requires planning, and it may be useful to involve potential users in planning and implementing the research and the dissemination (National Institute on Disability and Rehabilitation Research 2001).

Chapter summary

This chapter has described a research process suited to the majority of health-related qualitative research projects. The research process described was broken down into stages. The first stage requires a researcher to identify a research problem and develop a preliminary question (or set of questions). During this stage, their priority lies in finding a problem that captures their imagination and is also considered sufficiently important or interesting by others.

The next stage involves conducting a literature review and clarifying questions. During this stage a researcher is trying to familiarise themselves with what, where and how similar research has been conducted. They need to reflect on this research and their proposed research in a critical way. They may also need to develop or identify a suitable methodology and methods for their project.

The third stage of the research project is the design stage. Here a researcher is required to develop a research plan. This will entail becoming as clear as possible about what they are trying to achieve and how they will go about it. All researchers should get feedback from others during this stage.

The next stage in a research project involves thoughtful reflection about the ethical aspects of the research and gaining formal approval from an ethics committee or institutional research review board. Researchers should read guidelines on conducting ethical research and may need to alter their design in response to advice. Some projects then move to a stage where the researchers try to attract funding for the project.

The next and probably longest stage in the research process is data collection and analysis. This stage also involves the careful recording of research processes and findings. In a significant number of qualitative projects, data collection and analysis occur simultaneously. Researchers need to maintain their motivation and high research standards during this phase.

The final stage in the research process is the dissemination of results. Here the priority for researchers lies in letting others know about the research and its outcomes. Researchers may need to devise different dissemination strategies for different audiences.

Each stage of the process is important, and neglect during any stage can have negative repercussions for the overall success of the project. Thinking about the research process in stages makes the sheer volume of activity associated with a research project seem less overwhelming. It is also helpful to use the stages described in this chapter as a checklist when devising a timetable for a new research project. The case study below focuses on the data collection and analysis stages of a research project designed to evaluate an after-hours primary care service. The success of this evaluation reflects the careful planning conducted by the lead researcher, Lisa Crossland.

Case study: Evaluation of a longstanding after-hours primary care service

Ms Lisa Crossland, General Practice and Rural Health,
James Cook University, Australia

The word 'evaluation' carries with it many connotations and, for many people, equates to a 'score card' of results that rate how they have performed in rolling out a project, program or service. Prior to evaluating a longstanding after-hours primary medical service and specifically those factors that had contributed to the longevity of the service, there was much suspicion among the general practitioner members as to how we could possibly identify and explore the range of issues that had impacted on the service over the years, and if we were there to give them a 'mark out of ten'! Bearing these issues in mind and the complex nature of what we were trying to describe, the evaluation method was designed in consultation with the service representatives, as a qualitative study. The approach would allow us to identify and describe, in great detail, those factors that had contributed to the operational success of this after-hours service model across many years, including why the participating GPs were so happy to continue to provide after-hours calls in this context, despite the always fluctuating and often minimal payment for their time and effort.

During the evaluation, qualitative data was collected in four key stages. This enabled us to match issues and themes impacting on the longevity of service from a variety of sources. The four stages involved a comprehensive literature review to identify key themes and factors from national and international studies, a detailed 'map' of the development of the co-operative through a review of all materials relating to the operation and function of the service over time (these included minutes from meetings, protocols and guidelines, financial information and additional correspondence). Finally, we conducted in-depth semi-structured interviews with GPs, nursing and reception staff at the after-hours service and administered a patient survey which enabled us to explore many of the issues we identified during the review of materials.

The inclusion of the service participants at all stages in planning the methodological approach, and in particular the semi-structured interviews, was a key factor in the success of this evaluation. Close consultation enabled us to dispel many of the concerns about evaluation as a 'score card'. A shared understanding of the process of the qualitative approach with service members also facilitated open access to the full range of after-hours service materials on file, including all correspondence and minutes of meetings. This ultimately added to the depth and breadth of qualitative data available to us as evaluators.

The next challenge was in conducting in-depth, semi-structured and often time-consuming interviews with busy general practitioners. Previous studies have demonstrated that GPs are a group who do not respond well to long interviews, particularly those conducted via telephone during the day. Understandably, this impacts on busy consulting time and often leads to GPs dropping out of interviews before completion or refusing consent to participate from the outset. However, long interviews were a key approach in allowing us to explore the range of detail we had identified in our review of materials. We were worried no-one would consent to participate! The problem was solved with three key strategies. First, all interviews were conducted face-to-face, or postponed until the GP was available for a face-to-face meeting. This meant that we needed to ensure adequate funding was available for interviewer travel. Flexibility was needed in organising the meetings, but in order to keep within budget, clear and timely communication prior to the interview became paramount. Second, we provided clear information to all consenting GPs about the broad types of question they might be asked and the maximum time the interview would take. Finally, all interviews were conducted at the after-hours clinic during GP down time. If the GP was busy, we took the opportunity to talk with reception and nursing staff, where possible. The interviewer was committed to spending the entire evening (and often this meant continuing late into the night) at the service with the on-call GP, talking with them between consultations. This was the least disruptive way to complete the interviews and demonstrated a measure of commitment from the interviewer which was appreciated by the general practitioners. They responded by giving us thoughtful and reflective discussion on a range of issues and, once again, enhanced the richness of the data we gathered.

We could not control the fact that very sick patients would turn up during the course of an interview. Often the interviewer was required to break off mid-question, or the GP had to stop mid-sentence to attend to a patient. At this stage the interviewer simply moved back to the after-hours clinic tearoom, rewound the tape to the beginning of the discussion and replayed a short piece to assist in refocusing the GP and re-establishing the 'train of thought' once the interview recommenced.

While qualitative research methodology was the best approach for the subject we were exploring, it was certainly not the quickest or most practical method in relation to general practitioner participants. However, consultation and inclusion assisted in overcoming many suspicions about the approach, demonstrated understanding of the way interviews could be best conducted within a general practice context, and ensured that we gained the depth and richness of data to identify the key factors contributing to the longevity of this after-hours primary care service.

Recommended reading

Creswell, J.W. 2003, *Research design: Qualitative, quantitative and mixed methods approaches*, Sage Publications, Thousand Oaks, California.

Glesne, C. & Peshkin, A. 1992, *Becoming qualitative researchers*, Longman, New York.

Lofland, J. & Lofland, L.H. 1984, *Analyzing social settings: A guide to qualitative observation and analysis*, 2nd edn, Wadsworth, Belmont.

Maxwell, J. 1996, *Qualitative research design: An interactive approach*, Sage Publications, Thousand Oaks, California.

Morse, J.M. & Field, P.A. 1996, *Nursing research: The application of qualitative approaches*, Chapman & Hall, London.

Punch, K.E. 1998, *Introduction to social research: Quantitative and qualitative approaches*, Sage Publications, London.

three
RESEARCH DESIGN AND RIGOUR

Good researchers want to design projects that will be taken seriously and produce trustworthy data. In quantitative research this is achieved by following clearly established procedures to ensure rigour. However, in a qualitative research project the guidelines for designing a rigorous and therefore trustworthy project are less clear-cut. This ambiguity is a reflection of several issues. First, it is well recognised that applying the traditional scientific measures of rigour, such as objectivity, reliability and validity, to qualitative research is inappropriate (Blaikie 1993; Patton 1990:460). As explained in Chapter One, the fundamental differences between qualitative and quantitative research mean that the two approaches should not be judged against each other, nor the same measures used to evaluate them both.

The second hurdle to establishing straightforward criteria for designing a trustworthy qualitative project is the enormous diversity within qualitative research and, consequently, the differing opinions about what constitutes 'good' research (Denzin & Lincoln 1994; Glesne & Peshkin 1992). Researchers working within different qualitative theoretical frameworks often disagree with each other. Because of this, many writers argue that the quality of a researcher's work should only be judged using the measures appropriate to their particular research methodology (Blaikie 1991; Grbich 1999; Hammersly 1992). There has also been a tendency for qualitative researchers to actively resist attempts to standardise or evaluate their work via checklists or guidelines. While this issue is directly related to the difficulties associated with producing a checklist suitable to all types of qualitative research, a distrust of guidelines is also a reflection of the way that qualitative researchers tend to value artfulness, flexibility, creativity and serendipity (Barbour 2001; Sandelowski 1993:1).

Nevertheless, conducting qualitative social research is a skill with recognised techniques and methodologies. As such it is possible to give advice about how trustworthy and dependable qualitative projects can be designed. Without doubt, a thoughtful and carefully designed qualitative study will produce more robust and interesting results than one designed poorly. Furthermore, a commitment to flexibility and an acceptance of methodological plurality should not be used as an excuse for poor scholarship or slapdash design (Cheek 2004; Seale 1997). Silbey (2003) explains that the flexible and iterative nature of qualitative research should not preclude its capacity to be disciplined or systematic. She argues that a failure to develop an appropriate research design or to explain clearly how decisions were made about research design can be misinterpreted by others as simply 'making do' (2003:1). This reflects poorly on qualitative research in general and is therefore to be avoided:

> When done well, qualitative . . . health research has the ability to describe in depth the experiences of people's lives and the social contexts that strengthen, support or diminish health. It has the ability to humanise the research process and to lead to context specific strategies for individual and collective change. But, when poorly done, qualitative research at best confirms the fast-held beliefs of number crunchers and at worst provides misleading or sometimes harmful interpretations about the research subject's experiences. (Gifford 1996:58)

This chapter is focused on research design issues that were not covered adequately in the two previous chapters. These are rigour, strategies for improving the perceived rigour of a project, reflexivity, developing a qualitative methodology, and selecting appropriate qualitative data collection methods. The chapter closes with a case study from Annette Street and Amanda Hordern. Both of these researchers work in a school of nursing, and their case study reflects the high quality of qualitative research conducted within the nursing field. The authors describe developing a qualitative methodology for a research project investigating issues of sexuality and intimacy in cancer and palliative care.

Rigour in qualitative research

In quantitative research such as statistical and experimental studies, the term 'rigorous' is used to describe study designs that are valid and reliable. Validity refers to the extent to which a test or instrument measures what it claims to measure. This can also be explained as a concern with how accurately the research data reflects 'reality'. The term 'reliability' refers to the consistency of the research findings (Rice & Ezzy 1999:30; Sandelowski 1993). If a study can be repeated and obtain similar or identical results, it is assumed that the results are an accurate reflection of an external reality. Validity and reliability in quantitative research are achieved through the application of strict rules related to issues such as sampling, measurement instruments, statistical methods and the statistical power of the data analysis.

In contrast, qualitative researchers assume that to some extent what is perceived as reality is socially constructed and that the production of research results is a constructive and interactive process involving participants and researchers. Snadden (2001:1099), for example, asserts 'what is held to be true in one setting may be interpreted differently in another due to less definable issues such as culture and beliefs'. Accordingly, the traditional meanings of rigour as described above are difficult to use when conducting qualitative research. However, many qualitative researchers (particularly those working in the health arena) do assume that insights from qualitative research should reflect events and states of affairs that occur in people's lives (Hammersly 1992; Seale 1997). From this perspective of 'subtle realism', qualitative researchers want to design projects able to 'represent reality rather than to attain truth' (Mays & Pope 2000:51). As such, a rigorous qualitative study will address questions such as 'does the data appear to be accurately capturing the phenomena?' or 'what approach to sampling will suit this study?' (Denzin 1997). It will also require an intent to conduct a balanced and transparent analysis. Issues of validity are consequently seen as complex and ambiguous. Researchers want their research to represent the experiences or behaviours of participants in an accurate fashion, and to document their own biases and assumptions, so that the impact of these on their interpretations can be evaluated by the reader (Grbich 1999:62).

> When validation is viewed as a culturally and historically situated social process, both the experimentalist and interpretivist can be recognised as relying on contextually grounded linguistic and interpretive practices rather than on rules assumed to be sufficiently abstract and universal for every project. Trustworthiness becomes a matter of persuasion whereby the scientist is viewed as having made those practices visible and therefore audible. (Sandelowski 1993:2)

Lincoln and Guba (1985) outline several alternative criteria for rigour in qualitative research. These have since been used by other researchers and presented in qualitative textbooks (Hamberg et al. 1994). These indicators are credibility, dependability, confirmability and transferability. Credibility corresponds to a degree with notions of internal validity in traditional research (Hamberg et al. 1994:177). The credibility of a study is assessed by examining the findings and interpretations. If the reader considers that they represent some type of 'truth', they are deemed to be credible. The dependability of a research project is related to issues such as suitability of methods, and transparency of methods and analysis. A researcher should provide a clear account of the research process, allowing the reader to judge the dependability of the research.

Confirmability is a complex indicator. It refers to the importance of some degree of neutrality in research and establishes that the researcher has tried to avoid distorting the reality they are describing. Confirmability is often achieved by researchers conducting a reflexive analysis, describing the analytic process and by including large amounts of data in any written reports. This enables other researchers to 'judge findings and results as reasonable by looking into [the] data' (Hamberg et al. 1994:179). Transferability is the final criteria. To my mind it is one of the most useful indicators outlined by Lincoln and Guba. The results from qualitative research are rarely generalisable. To be generalisable, quantitative projects require significant statistical power and large, often randomised samples. However, the results from qualitative research are derived from relatively small purposeful samples and presented as interpretation and description. Therefore, they cannot be described as generalisable. Nevertheless, the results from qualitative research may be transferable. They should be understandable by others and recognisable. If the study context, methods, sampling and results are clearly outlined, it is possible for the reader to decide if the results are relevant to other similar situations (Lincoln & Guba 1985).

These criteria for discussing qualitative rigour are useful for qualitative researchers at two different levels. First, they are useful at a conceptual level because they encourage new ways of thinking about rigour and quality in qualitative research. Second, they may be useful when writing about or discussing research because they provide terms to describe qualitative rigour. This is particularly helpful when describing your research in research plans, reports and other publications.

There are several strategies often advocated to increase the rigour of qualitative research (Appleton 1995; Hamberg et al. 1994; Kirk & Miller 1986). These are triangulation, respondent validation, purposeful sampling, transparency of methods and analysis and researcher reflexivity. The majority of researchers who write about these strategies emphasise that their use does not 'in itself confer rigour' (Barbour 2001:1115). To be effective, these techniques need to be 'embedded in a broader understanding of the rationale and assumptions behind qualitative research' (Barbour 2001:1115). They also need to be used appropriately as they are not suited to all types of qualitative methodology (in particular, some are less suited to projects with a postmodern methodology, where researchers assume that their analysis need not bear any resemblance to an underlying 'reality' and where multiplicity is valued). Each of these strategies will be discussed in detail later in this chapter.

While there is considerable debate about rigour in the literature surrounding qualitative research, it seems clear that qualitative researchers need to maintain a balance between aiming for 'clear understanding' of the techniques that can be used to produce trustworthy qualitative work and 'succumbing to the illusion of technique' where it is assumed that simply following the correct steps will produce quality qualitative research (Sandelowski 1993:1). From this standpoint, rigour is 'less about adherence to the letter of the rules and procedures than it is about fidelity to the spirit of qualitative work' (1993:2). For example, Rice and Ezzy (1999) in their chapter on notions of rigour in qualitative research, recommend that researchers conduct rigorous research by taking a whole-picture approach to their project. They discuss rigour in relation to theory use, data collection procedures, analysis, interpretation and ethics. It follows that developing an appropriate methodology, selecting suitable data collection methods, conducting a reflexive and theoretically informed analysis and remaining aware of ethical and political aspects of the project are all related to rigour. Drawing on this perspective, I have developed the following list of suggestions for a rigorous qualitative project:

1 Begin with the researcher(s) familiarising themselves with writings and ideas underpinning qualitative methodologies and the particular problem/issue under study. (Note that in grounded theory, it is considered important to approach the study without established knowledge about the phenomena under study. This is because in grounded theory, a researcher avoids starting with existing theories. Instead, they study human experience and inductively extrapolate a theory.)

2 Have a researcher(s) who explicitly acknowledges the assumptions and ideas underpinning their research in their writing and analysis and who applies a critical gaze to their own interpretations and conclusions.

3 Ensure the research problem and research question(s) are suited to qualitative inquiry.

4 Make use of sampling strategies, methods of data collection and analysis appropriate to the research question and overall methodology.

Ensure that these are performed competently by researcher(s) and are described in sufficient detail that a reader can understand how data was collected and how it was analysed.

5 Provide adequate examples from the empirical data to support analytic claims and also include reference to other studies of the issue(s) being researched.

6 Be ethical. Insist on confidentiality and informed consent to participate in the research and address any other ethical issues (e.g. possible negative consequences for participants).

If we take a whole-picture approach to rigour, it is clear that many of the background issues a researcher needs to be aware of have already been discussed in the two earlier chapters of this book. These include the differences between qualitative and quantitative research, the role of theory in qualitative research and the importance of ethical considerations. Chapter Two explained the research process, outlining steps that need to be followed to bring a researcher to the point where they are able to design a rigorous study (e.g. conducting a literature review, identifying a research problem and clarifying research questions).

However, as mentioned above, other strategies are available that are often seen as increasing the rigour of a qualitative project. Their use appears to enhance the credibility of qualitative research and consequently the acceptability of qualitative research to funding bodies, some peer-reviewed journals and quantitative researchers (Rice & Ezzy 1999; Morse & Field 1996). This in turn may improve the likelihood that the study will successfully attract competitive grant funding and the results be published.

Techniques to improve rigour

The strategies of purposive sampling, triangulation, respondent validation (member checks), transparency of methods/analysis and researcher reflexivity, if used in a thoughtful and appropriate manner, may improve the quality of data and analysis of a research project. They may also make the results of your project more acceptable to others and therefore contribute to greater overall success.

Purposive sampling

Quantitative research studies generally rely on large randomly selected samples. 'The logic and power of probability sampling depends on selecting a truly random and statistically representative population that will permit confident generalisation from the sample to a larger population' (Patton 1990:169). Random sampling provides a sample of people along a continuum of varying quality on the topic of interest. In contrast, sampling in qualitative research is not concerned with producing findings that can be 'statistically generalised to the whole population' (Rice & Ezzy 1999:42). Instead the 'logic and power' of purposive sampling lie 'primarily in the quality of information obtained per sampling unit, as opposed to their number per se' (Sandelowski 1995:179). Qualitative analysis requires in-depth study and smaller samples than in quantitative research. Thus random sampling is not appropriate for qualitative studies.

However, this should not be interpreted as meaning the characteristics of research participants are unimportant or that research should involve any participants who are easy to include in the study (convenience sampling). Instead, sampling in qualitative research should be purposive. That is, it should aim at identifying and including in the study those information-rich cases that will provide a 'full and sophisticated under-standing of the phenomena under study' (Rice & Ezzy 1999:42). This will involve careful consideration of the aims of the study and thoughtful decision making about the desired range, characteristics and numbers of research participants (or other data sources). Judging the appropriate size of the sample in a qualitative project is relative. A sample should be neither too large nor too small in order to address the research questions (Sandelowski 1995:180). For example, an overly large sample will work against claims to have conducted a highly detailed analysis. An overly small sample could indicate that the researcher stopped their sampling prematurely. It is all related to the scope and purpose of the research project and the questions(s) being addressed. Some qualitative projects could have a sample of one and be quite valid, such as a qualitative case study focused on one person (Ruckdeschel et al. 1994). Barbour describes purposive sampling in the following terms:

> Purposive (or theoretical) sampling ... offers researchers a degree of control rather than being at the mercy of any selection bias inherent in pre-existing groups (such as clinical populations). With purposive sampling, researchers deliberately seek to include 'outliers' conventionally discounted in quantitative approaches. It allows for deviant cases to illuminate through juxtaposition, those processes and relations that routinely come into play. (Barbour 2001:1115)

There are numerous different methods of purposive sampling in qualitative research. Patton (1990:170–6) outlines many of these, as do Rice and

Ezzy (1999:43–6). For example, extreme case, or deviant case, sampling focuses on unusual or special cases (Patton 1990:170).

Intensity sampling also requires that the researcher select cases they consider to be information-rich. Unlike extreme case or deviant case sampling, however, they do not select unusual cases. Instead, 'using the logic of intensity sampling, one seeks excellent or rich examples of the phenomena under interest' (Patton 1990:171).

The strategy of maximum variability sampling aims at 'capturing and describing the central themes or principal outcomes that cut across a great deal of the participant or program variation' (Patton 1990:172).

In direct contrast to maximum variation sampling, homogenous sampling focuses on a 'particular subgroup in depth' (Patton 1990:173).

In typical case sampling, the researcher selects one or more 'typical' cases. This method requires considerable insider knowledge to enable the identification of such cases. Cases can act as 'qualitative profiles'. 'The purpose of a qualitative profile of one or more typical cases is to describe and illustrate what is typical to those unfamiliar with the program' (Patton 1990:173). Patton uses the example of selecting a typical village in a study of development projects in the Third World (1990:174).

In a critical case sampling strategy, the researcher selects cases that 'can make a point quite dramatically or are, for some reason, particularly important in the scheme of things' (1990:174). In keeping with this aim, the researcher chooses a research site or group of participants that will 'yield the most information and have the greatest impact on the development of knowledge' (1990:174).

Chain, or snowball, sampling is a method often used by researchers to locate important and information-rich cases (Lofland & Lofland 1984). The researcher asks key informants to suggest places or people to include in the study. Snowball sampling is frequently used in field-based studies as each participant can be asked to suggest a new person to be interviewed. 'Those people or events recommended as valuable by a number of different informants take on a special importance' (Patton 1990:176).

In criterion sampling, the researcher establishes a pre-determined criterion of importance. This could be males who attend a hospital outpatient clinic, with a diagnosis of testicular cancer who receive radiation therapy, for example. 'The point of criterion sampling is to be sure to understand cases that are likely to be information rich because they may reveal major system weaknesses and become targets of opportunity for program or system improvement' (Patton 1990:177).

The most crucial aspect of purposive sampling in qualitative research is that the researcher describes and justifies how decisions about sampling were made, why they were made and how the strategy was operationalised. They should also remember to carry their sampling strategy into the analysis of data. Barbour (2001) makes the point that in truly purposive sampling, simply mentioning the sampling strategy in the methods section of a research report is insufficient. Researchers also need to discuss the research findings in relation to the project sample; for example, discussing patterns in the data in terms of the characteristics of the research participants. Explaining how themes or meanings varied across a sample and discussing outlying cases will allow a researcher to 'illuminate subtle but potentially important differences' (2001:1116).

Triangulation

Combining different sampling strategies, methods, analysis approaches, and/or qualitative and quantitative research approaches in the same research project is know as triangulation (Denzin 1970:298; Meijer et al. 2002). It is a flexible technique as researchers can triangulate in one aspect of the project or across several. For example, combining different methods (often quantitative and qualitative) allows researchers to compare the consistency of their data. Combining multiple sources of data in the same project allows researchers to compare their data over time or to compare different types of data that may reflect different aspects of the project. Examples are comparing interview data with observational data, or focus group data with documents. Kimchi et al. (1991) provide definitions for six different types of triangulation. They draw on Denzin (1989) and review 319 qualitative research articles published in nursing journals between 1986 and 1987. These are summarised below.

Theory triangulation

Assessing the utility of competing theories through research. This is often achieved by using two or more competing theories in a single study.

Data triangulation

Using multiple data sources to obtain diverse views about the topic.

Methods triangulation

Using two or more methods in a study. Triangulation may occur within methods (e.g. using different types of data) and between different methods (e.g. comparing observation and interview data).

Investigator triangulation

Using two or more researchers with divergent backgrounds and disciplinary expertise. Each investigator plays an important role in the project with the aim of comparing or neutralising their differences.

Multiple triangulation

Using more than one type of triangulation within the same research project or to investigate the same event.

Analysis triangulation

Using more than one approach to analysis to analyse the same set of data.

Using more than one type of qualitative analysis can be a complicated form of triangulation; however, it also has great potential in some projects (Begley 1996). Examples are using a content analysis and an iterative thematic analysis in the same project or examining a particular research problem using a sociological theory and a theory from psychology.

Triangulation using multiple researchers also appears to be gaining in popularity in evaluation and health-related research (Patton 1990:468; Armstrong et al. 1997). Investigator triangulation using multiple researchers can be achieved in several different ways. In some projects, the researchers work together as a group; for example, coding transcripts and reading and reflecting on field notes (Douglas 1976). This approach is often used in ethnographic studies. Alternatively, the researchers can work independently, and the results of their analyses are later compared or an external person is used to review the coding and interpretations of others and comment on them (Freeman & Sweeney 2001; Daly et al. 1992).

However, it must be recognised that the use of multiple analysts for the purpose of comparison is problematic. The technique appeals strongly to quantitative researchers who see it as a way of circumventing the personal biases of investigators (Kimchi et al. 1991:365–6). However, this viewpoint assumes that there is 'fixed point or superior explanation' (Barbour 2001:1117). Such a viewpoint is not appropriate in qualitative research where the 'existence of multiple views of equal validity' are recognised (2001:117). Therefore, if the use of multiple researchers working independently at analysing the same data appeals to you, it is extremely important to clarify your expectations before you start. For example, are you expecting the multiple researchers to identify the same codes or themes in a transcript or are you simply hoping that multiple researchers will help your study to produce a more complex, wide-ranging analysis? An investigation of the technique by Armstrong et al. (1997) found a degree of concordance among six researchers asked to independently analyse focus group data at the level of 'themes within a wider framework' (1997:605). However, the researchers varied in how they packaged and expressed the themes. Different researchers are unlikely to produce the same results.

Methods triangulation and the comparison of qualitative and quantitative data for the purpose of validation has also been criticised (Morse 1994; Sandelowski 1993; Vidich & Lyman 1994). Pointing to the differences between qualitative and quantitative research, these authors conclude that results cannot be compared for the purpose of cross-checking (Blaikie 1991; Kelle 2001). Furthermore, many researchers consider that the assumptions underlying qualitative research do not readily support attempts to compare results from different qualitative methods (Armstrong et al. 1997:605). 'Research methods are not neutral tools that will produce the same results, regardless of the method' (Rice & Ezzy 1999:38).

As a result of these and other criticisms, the traditional use of triangulation (to compare the results from different methods or strategies with the aim of increasing the internal validity of a project) has been problematised. Researchers using triangulation for this purpose need to be clear about why they consider this to be appropriate in their project and to be able to demonstrate that their use of triangulation is congruent with their chosen methodology. Many researchers now prefer to use triangulation to develop a fuller, more complex picture of the problem or phenomenon under study rather than as a way of cross-checking, or validation. From this viewpoint, triangulation is conceived as a way of providing complementary perspectives and increasing the 'comprehensiveness' of qualitative research (Richardson 1991; Barbour 2001). Such an objective is congruent with the majority of qualitative methodologies.

Respondent validation

Respondent validation is a technique where transcripts or the results from a preliminary data analysis are shown to research participants. It is also termed 'member checking' (Morse & Field 1996). The opinions of the research participants about the accuracy of the transcripts or analysis are then incorporated into the study findings and a second round of analysis. The principal aim of this method is to 'establish the degree of correspondence between' the researcher's views and those of the research participants (Mays & Pope 2000:51). Researchers using respondent validation also hope that the method will help them to answer the questions, 'Do the findings of the study make sense? Are they credible to the people we study and to our readers? Do we have an authentic portrait of what we are looking at?' (Miles & Huberman 1994:278). This technique is clearly associated with two distinct themes within qualitative research. The first is a desire to accurately portray the experiences and viewpoints of research participants. This aim is associated with realist qualitative research traditions, such as ethnography. Respondent validation clearly presupposes that accuracy is a desirable and achievable aim. The second theme relates to the participatory aspects of qualitative perspectives, such as action research. Involving research participants in analysis and interpretation may increase their engagement with the research. This aspect of respondent validation makes it a popular technique among ethics committees and groups with an interest in consumer representation in research. Providing participants with an opportunity to challenge the interpretations of researchers is also likely to benefit researchers and assist with the production of quality analyses. Researchers do not have to agree with the participants but they should integrate their feedback into the analyses and discuss their views in any reports about the research (Lincoln & Guba 1985). For example, Nick Fox included feedback from surgeons about his analysis in his book *The Social Meaning of Surgery* (1992).

Respondent validation should not be used in an unthinking or uncritical manner (Atkinson 1997). The opinions of research participants cannot be taken to represent any type of authenticity. Furthermore, individual participants may have difficulties when asked to comment on analyses that present abstract statements about structural and cultural issues that do not reflect their individual experiences (Mays & Pope 2000:51). In addition, if participants perceive the researcher's analyses as unflattering towards them, they are unlikely to agree with them (Sandelowski 1993:5; Fox 1992).

Respondent validation is problematic in qualitative research perspectives that view participant accounts as narratives. Ideas, memories and narratives shift in the telling and retelling. Accordingly, while the researcher may gain insight from asking participants to comment on their previous statements, this process may not be related to checking for accuracy. 'Researchers employing member checking are always obligated to ensure that any correction of contents or feeling tone is warranted as a correction and not as a new story that must be analysed for its meaning in relation to other stories' (Sandelowski 1993:5). Furthermore, researchers utilising respondent validation as a way of checking for accuracy need to be aware of the many different functions that partic-ipants' accounts can fulfil. These may include, 'normative statements (what people say should be the case), narrative reconstructions (biographically specific reinterpretations of what has happened in the past), and actual practices (what really happens)' (Lambert & McKevitt 2002:211).

Transparency of methods and analysis

A rigorous qualitative study should clearly describe how the research was conducted, how and why participants were selected, what methods were used and how the analysis was conducted (procedural rigour). This allows readers to judge for themselves the suitability of the research design for addressing the research question. In many studies it is also appropriate to include information about how access was obtained and how many people were approached but refused to participate (Rice & Ezzy 1999:36; Altheide & Johnson 1994:493). In studies making use of interview, focus group and field data, it is vital to include sufficient examples of this data (e.g. quotations) to support analytical statements and claims. Any discussion of the analysis and results should also include mention of negative cases, outliers and alternative explanations. A detailed account of data collection and analysis serves to highlight the creative and interpretive nature of qualitative research:

> The qualitative researcher has an obligation to be methodical in reporting sufficient details of data collection and the processes of analysis to permit others to judge the quality of the resulting product . . . It is important to report what alternative classification schemes, themes and explanations are considered and 'tested' during data analysis. This demonstrates intellectual integrity and lends considerable credibility to the final set of findings . . . (Patton 1990:462)

While triangulation and respondent validation are best suited to projects conducted within a realist tradition, transparency of methods and analysis is a technique associated with rigour that is suited to all types of qualitative research. Even projects not bound by the traditional expectations associated with scientific inquiry (e.g. projects with post-modern and some feminist methodologies) require a scholarly attention to detail and a clearly articulated method and methodology (Cheek 2004; Gifford 1996). The key aspect of transparency of methods and analysis is that the researcher includes sufficient detail in any reporting of their work for the readers to judge the quality of the study for themselves.

Reflexivity

Reflexivity 'implies that the researcher understands that he or she is part of the social world(s) that he or she investigates' (Berg 2004:154). Being reflexive means that a researcher aims to achieve 'explicit, self aware analysis of their own role' (Finlay 2002:531). Being a reflexive researcher is another way of conducting rigorous qualitative research that is suited to all types of qualitative study. While reflexivity came into prominence though ethnographic, feminist, postmodern and poststructural research, the process is now valued across the various qualitative methodologies (Rice & Ezzy 1999:40–1).

Conducting research in a reflexive manner requires recognition that a researcher becomes part of the group or setting they are studying. It also involves awareness of the impact of the researcher's own personal characteristics, training and beliefs on the development of research questions, data collection, analysis and the ensuing results. Being reflexive helps a researcher to conduct quality research in a number of different ways.

Reflexivity encourages honest consideration about a researcher's role in their project (Shacklock & Smyth 1998). This may help them to improve their study design and the way they conduct themselves over the course of the project (particularly in relation to research participants). Reflexivity also assists researchers to question their own assumptions and interpretations (and those of their research participants and fellow researchers). As reflexivity should be carried into the written reports of the project, the stance should place these assumptions within the view of people reading about the research. Patton (1990:472) suggests that in recognising that a researcher is 'the instrument in qualitative inquiry' and in the interests of establishing researcher credibility, a qualitative report should include information about the researcher(s). For example, their age, sex, training and background, relationship (if any) to the research participants and/or funding bodies and any personal connections with the research topic. Many other writers also recommend that qualitative research reports use the pronoun 'I' when describing the experiences or interpretations of the researcher(s). In this way a researcher can assert their 'ownership and responsibility' for their views (Berg 2004:156).

> Reflexivity further implies a shift in the way we understand data and their collection. To accomplish this, the researcher must make use of an internal dialogue that repeatedly examines *what the researcher knows* and *how the researcher came to know this*. The reflexive ethnographer does not merely

report *findings as facts* but actively constructs interpretations of experiences in the field and then questions how these interpretations actually arose. (Berg 2004:154)

An article that demonstrates a reflexive approach to qualitative research is Hamberg et al. (1994). Their study involved family doctors interviewing 20 female patients. They were acutely aware of the complexities associated with gathering and interpreting interview data and wrote extensively about this. For example:

To conclude, credibility in data collection depended on the degree of closeness and mutual respect established, the interviewing skills of the researcher, motives and strategies of participating women, the impact of the fact that researchers were also physicians and finally, how the power structure of the patient–doctor relationship influenced the outcome. (Hamberg et al. 1994:178)

Developing a methodology

I have touched upon the importance of methodology in a qualitative research project many times already in this chapter and earlier chapters of this book. This issue is explained here in more detail because a thoughtful and appropriate methodology is necessary for a rigorous qualitative project (Rice & Ezzy 1999; Maxwell 1996; Kirk & Miller 1986). Methodology is a term used to explain the justification given by the researcher for why particular methods of data collection and analysis have been selected and are appropriate. Where research methods describe how you plan to go about collecting and making sense of data, a methodology describes and justifies why you have chosen this particular research method (Rice & Ezzy 1999:10).

As described in Chapter One, some qualitative projects (particularly those conducted for applied research) can be seen as largely method-driven. That is, the researcher makes little explicit use of theory when justifying their methods or interpreting their results. However, most qualitative research projects justify the choices of method by being located within a particular theoretical or methodological approach (Patton 1990). The theoretical underpinnings of a research project are extremely powerful. They shape the way 'practitioners and researchers collect and interpret evidence' (Alderson 1998:1007).

The following examples of theoretical approaches from philosophy and the social sciences illustrate the associations between particular theoretical perspectives and certain qualitative research methods. After reading it, you may be able to place research you have read or are thinking of conducting within one or more of the perspectives. Many other theoretical perspectives are taken up by qualitative researchers. However, all of those listed below have been widely used in academic and applied qualitative research and will be easy to follow up in other books and journals. It is good to recognise that although theoretical perspectives are often described as distinct, in reality the distinctions between different theories and approaches are often ambiguous. The various perspectives have developed over time and each builds on the other. Many individual writers and theorists are described as advocating or representing more than one perspective. Furthermore, individual researchers often draw on more than one theoretical framework in their work.

Ethnography

Ethnographies aim to study and describe a culture. In this context, the term 'culture' can refer to ethnic groups, a geographical location, professional groups, other groups and organisations. In other words, the culture being studied could range from Hmong people living in southern California to a ward in an Australian public hospital. Traditionally, ethnographies were conducted in an attempt to understand exotic and unfamiliar places and people. More recently ethnographies have been used to view the familiar with fresh eyes. Ethnography is an approach developed within anthropology but also used extensively in sociology, nursing, public health, geography and primary care (Hill 2003; Whittaker 1996). For example, Varcoe et al. (2003) used ethnography to explore the dynamics of healthcare relationships in different contexts. Kaufert and O'Neill (1993) used an ethnographic approach to explore the differing understandings of risk related to childbirth held by clinicians, epidemiologists and Inuit women.

The data and analysis produced in ethnographic studies is often described as 'thick description' due to a focus on detailed descriptions of people, places, understandings and things. Ethnographic studies make use of pre-existing understandings and the theoretical knowledge of the researcher (Denzin 1997; Spradley 1979). Ethnographic researchers try to gain an in-depth understanding of a culture, often over a long period of time. There are several different types of ethnographic study. These include classical ethnography, critical ethnography and auto-ethnography (Grbich 1999:167). Ethnographies are sometimes described as 'fieldwork' studies. This is because the data collection methods associated with ethnography all involve the researcher entering the field (research setting) and exploring the culture via interviews and participant observation techniques. Participant observation where a researcher conducts observation 'while participating in the study community' allows researchers doing an ethnographic study to learn about local context (Lambert & McKevitt 2002:211). Researchers may also collect textual data and objects such as clothing, tools and art.

Lambert and McKevitt argue that ethnographies informed by anthropological knowledge have considerable benefits for health research because they allow for informal data gathering which in turn allows researchers to explore the differences between 'what people say, think and do' and to avoid inaccurate generalisations (2002:210). Learning about a culture can also assist with understanding issues such as the context-dependent nature of conceptions of the body or the meanings given to physical symptoms (Kleinman 1988:13).

Phenomenology

Researchers using a phenomenological approach are interested in people's experiences in regard to the issue under study and how they interpret their experiences. Phenomenology is considered to be both a philosophical perspective and a methodological approach. Phenomenological inquiry questions 'the structure and essence of experience' (Patton 1990:69). Research drawing on the phenomenological tradition relies heavily on in-depth interviewing and diary entries, as these are seen as the most reliable sources of information about the meanings people give to their experiences. 'Phenomenologists study situations in the everyday world from the viewpoint of the experiencing person' (Becker 1992:7). As an approach, phenomenology has been particularly popular in nursing and psychological research where researchers have investigated the experience of illness and 'the relationship between the self, identity and the body' (Nettleton 1995:108). One such example is Corin and Lauzon's (1992) study of the experience of living with schizophrenia. Research projects conducted using a phenomenological perspective aim to develop a narrative account ending with theoretical propositions.

Symbolic interactionism and grounded theory

Symbolic interactionism is a theoretical approach focused on discovering how people define reality. The key assumptions underpinning symbolic interactionism are that human actions are a result of the meanings they give to things (such as words, objects, procedures etc); meaning arises out of social interaction; people modify their meanings through an interpretive process (Blumer 1969:2). In other words, 'Meanings are continually created, recreated and moderated in interaction' (Rice & Ezzy 1999:17).

While most empirical qualitative research is indirectly influenced by symbolic interactionism, the most direct link between the approach and contemporary qualitative methodologies is 'grounded theory' (Strauss & Corbin 1990; Glaser & Strauss 1968). Grounded theory is an inductive technique that involves highly descriptive accounts of social interaction and a focus on the meanings and interpretations of research participants. Grounded theory originated in 1967 with the researchers Glaser and Strauss. They developed the approach as a way of 'formalising the operations needed to develop theory from empirical data' (Green 1998:1064). Since that time, grounded theory has been adapted and refined by many other researchers (e.g. Charmaz 1983; 1990; Corbin & Strauss 1990; Glaser 1978; Martin & Turner 1986; Dey 1999). While there is ongoing debate about what actually is meant by grounded theory, I have summarised my own interpretation of the key tenets of grounded theory based closely on Dey (1993, 1999) and Strauss and Corbin (1994, 1998). This is outlined below:

- Generating or discovering theory derived from data acquired through fieldwork interviews, observations and documents. 'Theories are interpretations made from given perspectives as adopted or researched by researchers' (Strauss & Corbin 1994:171). Theory 'consists of plausible relationships proposed among concepts and sets of concepts . . . [it] is conceptually dense – that is, it deals with many conceptual relationships' (Strauss & Corbin 1994:278).
- Setting aside (at least initially) theoretical ideas, such as those acquired by reading other research and sociological theory, to allow a substantive theory to emerge from the data. Thus 'theories are always traceable to that data that gave rise to them . . . in which the analyst is also a crucially significant interactant' (Strauss & Corbin 1994:278–9).
- Focusing on individuals and the way they interact in relation to the phenomena under study. In grounded theory, the voices of research participants should be central (Dey 1993:1). This implies a focus on the micro level, such as the stories, narratives and other strategies that participants have used to achieve meaning. However, many researchers have broken away from a 'primary focus on micro phenomena' to also address 'historical matters of macro structure as a means of enriching research' (Layder 1993:68).
- Systematic data analysis which begins with the initial collection of data and involves identifying categories and connecting them. The process of

'coding' is a key feature of grounded theory. This process involves 'open coding', 'axial coding' and 'selective coding' (Dey 1999:259). Also associated with the analysis is the presentation of information about the process of analysis in the written report of the research. The 'transparency' achieved allows for comparison and verification. 'Those who use grounded theory accept responsibility for their interpretive roles. They do not believe it sufficient merely to report or give voice to the viewpoints of the people, groups or organisations being studied. Researchers assume the further responsibility of interpreting what is observed, heard or read' (Strauss & Corbin 1994:160).

- Reporting the resulting theory in a narrative framework as a set of propositions. This framework usually involves the use of excerpts from the interview transcripts (or other types of data) presented in an embedded manner with the researcher's interpretations (Dey 1999:2).

A recent review of qualitative research published in medical journals focused on oncology and palliative care found that grounded theory was the 'most employed methodological approach' (Borreani et al. 2004:7). For example, Kathy Charmaz used a grounded theory approach to explain how participants in her study managed living with a chronic illness (Charmaz 1990 and 1991). Shepard et al. (1999) used the approach to build a theoretical framework to explain the characteristics of expert physical therapy practitioners.

While there are many reasons for the popularity of grounded theory among health researchers, three factors stand out. First, grounded theory places great emphasis on 'the perspectives and voices of the people [being studied]' (Strauss & Corbin 1994:160). This is why the approach appeals to researchers who want to learn about the phenomena under study from the perspective of the research participants. Second, unlike many other qualitative approaches, grounded theory has a clearly outlined 'how-to-do' framework. Grounded theory has quite prescriptive data collection and analysis techniques aimed at producing a theory explaining the phenomena or issues under study. Consequently, a researcher can follow concrete steps as outlined by key texts that describe how to collect and analyse data. This is appealing to many qualitative researchers and to researchers familiar with the structured research designs used in quantitative research. Third, the explicitly inductive 'grounded' nature of the approach means that grounded theory research projects are rarely seen as being aligned with any particular political or ideological perspective.

Feminist theories

Feminist theories have been highly influential in the field of qualitative research. While there is enormous variability among feminist theories, a concern with gender and an acceptance that women are oppressed tend to be common across the field (Roberts 1989). Methodologies influenced by feminist theories emphasise the use of research methods that 'examine the experience and subjectivity of the person being studied' (Rice & Ezzy 1999:18). Feminist theories have also changed the ways that researchers think about qualitative research by drawing attention to the political nature of research and the potential for research to be exploitative or to reinforce inequalities (Smith 1987). Consequently, researchers employing a feminist methodology tend to favour participatory, emancipatory and egalitarian research that includes reference to the researcher's role, position and emotions (Clough 1994). Qualitative researchers influenced by feminist theory and writings also tend to place considerable emphasis on ethical issues (Järviluoma et al. 2003). The data collection methods favoured in projects of this kind are those that facilitate involvement from research participants, such as participant observation, interviews and focus groups. Feminist researchers have also conducted qualitative research using documents. Examples include studies of how female bodies are represented in medical textbooks or in popular culture (Farran 1990; Martin 1987).

Participatory action research

Participatory action research (PAR), also described as action research, is not really a theory. It is better defined as an approach, method or 'tool' developed to assist researchers and research participants to work together during the research project with the aim of changing or improving a situation (Cohen et al. 1992). Nevertheless, PAR has achieved the status of a qualitative approach and is often used as a methodology in academic research and evaluation (Malterud 1995). The defining feature of PAR is:

> a dual commitment in action research to study a system and concurrently to collaborate with members of the system in changing it in what is together regarded as a desirable direction. Accomplishing this twin goal requires the active collaboration of researcher and client, and thus it stresses the importance of co-learning as a primary aspect of the research process. (O'Brian 1998:2)

In PAR, traditional distinctions between the researcher and research participants are deliberately broken down. In many projects, research participants are actively involved in developing research questions, designing the project, and gathering and analysing data. Data collection methods are those that support the aims of PAR, such as unstructured interviewing, focus groups and participant observation (Meyer & Bridges 1998). Action research is a popular methodological approach in nursing and education that has also been used extensively in health programs aimed at oppressed or marginalised people (Hart & Bond 1995; de Konig & Martin 1996:4; Meyer 2000).

Postmodernism and poststructuralism

Postmodernism is a term given to a group of writings and ideas that emphasise the uncertainty of knowledge. Researchers taking a postmodern stance tend to be 'skeptical about what truth is, what counts as knowledge, and who can determine the validity or worth of any enterprise' (Alderson 1998:1009). A postmodern approach stands in opposition to assumed certainty of scientific explanation. For example, postmodernists often question medical definitions of disease and the tools used to diagnose. This approach reveals 'medical facts' as socially constructed rather than as stable and objective representations of reality. Cheek (2000) provides the following statement about postmodern thought:

> It disavows the idea that human experience can be reduced to, and captured by grand or totalising theories. Rather postmodern thought emphasises the plural nature of reality, the multiple positions from which it is possible to view any aspect of reality including healthcare and the partial nature of any form of representation of reality that arises from any form of writing/speaking. (Cheek 2000:5)

Poststructural approaches have a great deal in common with postmodern thought. They also emphasise plurality and multi-vocality (Cheek 2000:6). However, poststructural approaches focus mainly on language as 'the place where social meanings are defined, constructed and contested' (Grbich 1999:50). Poststructuralist and postmodern writers both place importance on individual perspectives and are 'highly skeptical of explanations which claim to be valid for all groups, cultures, traditions or races' (Counterbalance Glossary 2005).

Postmodernism and poststructuralism are relative newcomers as methodological underpinnings for qualitative research. The theorists and researchers working in these areas first became prominent in the late 1970s and during the '80s. However, the philosophical influences behind post-structuralist and postmodern thought have a long history. These include phenomenology, symbolic interactionism, psychoanalysis/semiotics and literary theory (Kellehear 1993:28).

In relation to qualitative research, one of the hallmarks of postmodern and poststructural approaches is the way various proponents have challenged prevailing research practices. In particular, they have raised questions about the relationships between power and knowledge and challenged 'taken-for-granted' assumptions about research. For instance, when viewed from a poststructuralist approach, research questions are not 'found', instead they are 'produced' from a limited range of possible choices (Allen 2003).

Researchers drawing on poststructuralist and postmodern theory have often rejected – or are at least highly critical of – traditional expectations about how research should be conducted or what research results should look like (Kellehear 1993:28). Researchers working within these traditions also tend to value chaos, contradiction, complexity, multiplicity of perspectives and deconstruction (Grbich 1999:24). As a result, they often conduct innovative and challenging studies (Prus 1996; Faberman 1992).

The work of poststructuralist theorist Michel Foucault has been particularly influential in health-related qualitative research (Fox 1993; Foucault 1967). Foucault argued that discourses 'govern the variety of ways in which it is possible to talk about something and thus make it difficult, if not impossible to think and act outside them' (Allen 2003:18). Discourses stem from discursive practices – 'a delimitation of a field of objects, the definition of a legitimate perspective for the agent of knowledge and the fixing of norms for the elaboration of concepts and theories' (Foucault 1977:199).

Research influenced by Foucault emphasises the deconstruction of language and discourses (Cheek 2000:6). Researchers might explore, for example, the ways that language is used to talk about aspects of health or disease in medical case notes, medical textbooks, health promotion advertisements or newspaper articles (Tulloch 1992; Chapman 1994; Lupton 1995). This research method is often described as discourse analysis and has been well accepted among qualitative researchers working in health-related fields such as public health and nursing (Leishman 2003; Avdi et al. 2000).

Qualitative data collection methods

Research methods are the means by which new data is collected. All qualitative data collection methods involve collecting data in the form of words, talk, experiences and actions. Most involve some degree of interaction between researchers and research participants. The exception to this is documentary data. Another category of data collection methods is field-based methods, such as observation, participant observation and unstructured interviewing and those methods that involve collecting data in a largely created situation, such as semi-structured interviewing and focus groups. Qualitative methods are based on the assumptions expressed in qualitative methodologies. While these vary, they tend to be united in a belief that 'real and trustworthy knowledge is found by paying attention to what people say and do in specific circumstances' (Roberts & Taylor 1998:170).

As discussed in Chapter Two and earlier in this chapter, selecting the most appropriate methods of data collection is closely related to the research questions and the methodology for a project. Methods need to collect the type of data required to address research questions and to sit easily with the methodological assumptions underpinning the project (Morse & Fields 1996; Patton 1990:9). There are also a number of pragmatic considerations related to choosing data collection methods. For example, the methods chosen should suit the skills and attributes of the researcher(s) and their capacity in terms of time, equipment and administrative support. Qualitative data collection methods are dependent on the skills of the researcher. A skilled, thoughtful and conscientious researcher is far more likely to collect high-quality data than an unskilled, poorly prepared or careless one. While this holds true for all types of research, the largely interactive nature of qualitative research makes it particularly vulnerable in terms of the relationship between data quality and the attributes and skills of the researchers collecting the data (Berg 2004).

The next three chapters of this book discuss in detail the methods of observation, interviewing and focus groups. There are, however, many other methods of data collection used in qualitative research. A brief overview of the most frequently used methods follows.

Observation and participant observation

Observation is an unobtrusive method of data collection that involves watching, listening and recording social activity. Participant observation requires that the observer also participates to some extent. Their participation may range from merely speaking with research participants to becoming fully engaged in the observed activity. Observation has many advantages for qualitative researchers. These include seeing what is happening, rather than being told by others what happens (i.e. observing actual behaviour) and gaining social, cultural and environmental information. Participant observation allows researchers to learn about a setting or situation through their own experiences. It is also useful for building rapport and 'getting to know' research participants. An advantage shared by observation and participant observation is that very little equipment is required. A note pad should be all a researcher needs.

The principal disadvantage of observation and participant observation is a significant limitation in sample size. Only small numbers or participants can be observed at one time, and researchers are only able to observe for relatively short periods of time before becoming exhausted or needing to pause and take notes. Furthermore, focused observation is a highly skilled activity and not suitable for beginner researchers with no access to training in this method. With participant observation, recording data poses difficulties as the researcher may need to remove themself from the 'field'. Added to this, issues related to informed consent make this an ethically complex data collection method.

Interviewing

Interviewing involves speaking with research participants. The type of data collected is conversation between an interviewer and an interviewee(s). An interview is usually conducted between an interviewer and no more than two interviewees. There are at least three types of qualitative interview – the structured interview, the semi-structured interview and the unstructured interview. Unstructured interviews range from short informal conversations that occur during participant observation to lengthy in-depth interviews that may last for hours or even days. Interviews are probably the most widely used qualitative data collection method. They have a high degree of acceptability as a data collection method among researchers, research participants and the consumers of research (Borreani et al. 2004). Interviews have a number of advantages, including flexibility, the capturing of participants' own words and the opportunity they provide for researchers to spend time with participants. Interviews are also valuable in studies where the researcher wants to build a relationship with research participants. Semi-structured and unstructured interviews facilitate in-depth understanding. This degree of understanding of the participant's point of view cannot be achieved using any other data collection method. The main disadvantage of interviewing is that it is an extremely labour-intensive method, particularly if interviews are fully transcribed. They also require recording equipment and some training.

Focus groups

Focus groups are group discussions on a focused topic. A relatively new data collection technique, focus groups have been used by researchers working within and across a range of traditions and methodologies (Berg 2004). Focus group discussions are usually recorded and transcribed in ways very similar to interview data. Focus groups have many advantages. Unlike most interviews, they allow researchers to capture group interaction between research participants. While this will not be the same type of interaction found in 'natural' groups, it still allows researchers to learn about language, and about issues seen as important to the group, and to make use of interaction as a way of triggering discussion. Focus groups are frequently used in the early stages of a project to help the researcher gain an overview of an unfamiliar situation or participants' views. They are also a flexible data collection method. The disadvantages of focus groups include time constraints, limitations in the number of issues that can be discussed and problems associated with group interaction. Focus groups also pose ethical challenges related to confidentiality and anonymity. Furthermore, focus group moderation is a skilled activity, and the quality of data is directly related to the quality of the facilitation. Researchers can also experience difficulties in accessing recording equipment suited to focus group data.

Open-ended questionnaires

Open-ended questionnaires have no set response categories. Instead, research participants fill in their own responses in blank spaces; they may also attach additional pages if they want to make particularly long responses. The type of data collected is textual and is seen to reflect the views of those completing the questionnaire. While open-ended questionnaires are not suited for in-depth data, they have a major advantage for studies requiring larger numbers of research participants because they can be given to large numbers of people. Their open-ended nature overcomes the problem associated with standardised questionnaires where responses may reflect the researcher's viewpoint rather than that of the respondents. However, open-ended questionnaires are highly labour-intensive in terms of analysis, and this limits the total number of questionnaires that can be administered.

It can also be difficult to motivate research participants to take the time to complete them. Open-ended questionnaires are unsuited to research where participants are likely to have difficulties with writing or reading. In addition, participants may find completing the questionnaire difficult because they are unable to ask for clarification or to have questions explained. Researchers may find the results from open-ended questionnaires frustrating because they are unable to ask the respondents new or additional questions about the replies. As such they are a useful method to use prior to interviewing participants or designing focus groups. Open-ended questions can also be added to quantitative questionnaires.

Journaling

Diaries and journals are the source of subjective information and in some studies can replace interviews. Diaries completed by participants provide data that clearly represents what the participants thought was important about a given event or behaviour. In health-related research, diaries are often given to participants who are asked to record experiences, feelings about events, or concrete details about diet, medications etc. While diaries are usually handwritten they could also be completed on-line, or using digital recorders or tape recorders. Diaries are also kept by researchers during the research process and used during analysis to provide context and data that records the feelings and experiences of the researcher. Advantages of journaling include having data that has been recorded by participants themselves and overcoming to a degree the 'managed public performances' of interactive data collection methods (Grbich 1999:143). Other advantages include the value obtained when diary data can be compared with field data or other types of data (Mechanic 1989). Disadvantages include the need to analyse textual data as this is less commonly done in health research and many researchers are unfamiliar with techniques. There may also be difficulties associated with legibility, collecting diaries from participants and motivating participants to complete diary entries. Diaries that are completed by hand or on-line are unsuitable for studies where participants have trouble with reading or writing. This may be overcome if diaries are maintained in an audio format.

Other types of documentary and textual data

Qualitative research can make use of documentary and textual data other than diaries. This could include health promotion materials, medical case notes, x-rays, policy documents, historical records, books, photographs, films, magazines or appointment books (McClelland et al. 2000; Lupton 1994b). Documentary data has many advantages. It can be used to provide context to other types of qualitative data or used alone. It can often be collected without ethical approval and is an unobtrusive research method

(Kellehear 1993). Documentary data can be used to provide detail and context for other types of data or analysed in its own right, as in discourse analysis.

Chapter summary

This chapter has focused on topics and issues that are important when designing a qualitative research project. These are the issue of rigour and strategies for improving the perceived rigour of a project, developing a qualitative methodology and how the selection of qualitative data collection methods can be done appropriately. Designing a project is often exciting but also daunting. Most beginner researchers are worried about 'getting it wrong'. This concern stems from several factors: recognition that research should be conducted to the best of a researcher's ability because it is important and may impact on real people's lives, health and wellbeing as well as the professional reputation of the researcher; lessons learnt studying quantitative research and when learning critical appraisal skills where projects are expected to meet standardised criteria for 'good research'; and straightforward (and perfectly understandable) panic when confronted with the sheer volume of potential methodologies and methods associated with qualitative research.

My advice is to remain calm and keep your early research designs simple. Remember that qualitative research doesn't follow a simple recipe. Provided you think things through and are able to justify your choices then your design is probably a good one. It takes time to become an experienced and skilled researcher and as a beginner you should be seeking advice and guidance from others and reading as widely as possible (see the list of recommended readings at the end of this chapter). The following case study from Annette Street and Amanda Hordern will serve as a reminder of the enormous potential of qualitative research designs to develop knowledge that is appropriate to the discipline of nursing.

Case study: Getting started with a sexy research project
Professor Annette F. Street & Dr Amanda Hordern, La Trobe University and
Austin Health Clinical School of Nursing, Australia

Sex sells. Aspects of sexuality dominate the media. Being bombarded with these images, it could be confidently assumed that our society is open to many forms of intimacy and sexuality, yet it remains a taboo area in cancer and palliative care. Health professionals assume that their patients are too worried about their diagnosis and treatment options to be concerned about personal issues such as intimacy and sexuality. Therefore, it is usually only raised when a cancer diagnosis will impact on fertility or sexual function, and even then the consultation will use formal language such as erectile dysfunction that may leave the person confused as to what this means for them. We knew this was a problem because a large number of calls to the the Cancer Council helpline telephone service asked questions about sexuality.

A literature review provided little evidence that people with cancer had been asked what their concerns were and how they wanted them addressed. So we began to plan a study to investigate the issues around intimacy and sexuality in the largest cancer service in Australia. We wanted to explore meaning, but also to involve health professionals and patients in developing strategies that might guide practice.

In the context of nursing, qualitative research encourages the researcher to explore the health system, investigating health as the multidimensional and complex experiences of individuals, their families, social and cultural forces. When qualitative research illuminates the meanings and structures of everyday clinical practice, strategies can be developed so that qualitative research has the capacity to directly impact upon the experiences of health professionals and the patients in their care.

Before we firmed up our question and method we decided to discuss our ideas with the medical and nursing gatekeepers of the different clinical units. We spoke at a number of hospital forums about the proposed research, inviting staff to contribute to its design and to participate in it. We conducted informal discussions with nursing unit managers about the project over morning tea to obtain their input into the study design and recruitment decisions within the project. Helpful advice was provided about advertising the project and a comprehensive list of key contact people was compiled that aided recruitment.

In doing this we were aware that Amanda came to the research with a range of identities that intersected with the aims of the research. As a nurse counsellor at the Cancer Council Victoria, Amanda had been directly involved in extensive education, training and counselling programs for health professionals and patients in the area of cancer and palliative care. This placed Amanda as an 'insider' with nurses and other health professionals within the research project as she procured trust from gatekeepers and health professional participants throughout the research, and 'outsider' when it came to the specific political and economic culture of the hospital setting under study. Annette carried her own shifting subject positions into the context as a sociologist who teaches and researches primarily with doctors and nurses. Her appointment at the hospital meant that she had 'insider' status as part of the institutional context and 'outsider' status because of her professional status.

The first meeting with an oncologist was not so promising as he equated the terms 'sexuality' and 'intimacy' purely with sexual function and could not think of *'one patient who would want to or be capable of this level of discussion'*. Fortunately, other oncologists had more imagination and were supportive. However, speaking from their own experiences of drug trials, they suggested that we should develop our questions around a particular tumour stream, such as breast or prostate. We disagreed, but these discussions shaped our sampling frame. We decided to obtain sufficient numbers of patient interviews to provide participant representation from the top four cancers (breast, prostate, bowel and lung cancer). This would help with credibility (a political reason) and data saturation (a data credibility reason). A large or representative sample is not a usual concern of qualitative studies directed at exploring meaning, but we wanted to not only understand the key issues but also to develop possible change strategies.

It was time to make a final decision on our topic and method. Drawing on the writings of Anthony Giddens, we decided to undertake a *reflexive inquiry* to conduct a study that was responsive to the data that emerged from the field and that enabled us to work reflexively with the theory, emergent conceptualisations and expert advice in order to design a framework to improve practice. The study was entitled 'Issues of intimacy and sexuality in cancer and palliative care' and aimed at collecting interview data to be analysed in association with a textual analysis of national guidelines and feedback on our evolving findings from a range of sources. Therefore, the data for this project consisted of a total of 82 semi-structured interviews with 50 patients and 32 health professionals, textual analysis of 33 national and international clinical practice guidelines, the participant feedback from 15 patient and health professional educational forums, and reflective journaling throughout the research process.

The interview data were transcribed and imported into the NVivo computer package, along with the reflective journal, summaries of the relevant literature and Gidden's theoretical ideas, clinical practice guidelines (either directly or through linked documents) and the feedback from the forums. The reflexive nature of the project ensured that there was a deliberate and systematic use of researcher responses to the evolving data analysis and the structured responses of others to this data. This involved an exploration of our own attitudes and beliefs about patient issues of intimacy and sexuality throughout the reflexive inquiry and how these personal definitions impacted on the way we analysed the data throughout this research. Amanda become increasingly aware of how her definitions of patient sexuality and intimacy structured the ways in which she communicates with patients and health professionals at a clinical practice level.

All of this material was coded and categorised concurrently, and constantly refined over the period of the study. Each textual source was integrated with the others so that the key issues identified by the health professionals and patients became evident and a clusters of responses emerged along a continuum. We contrasted the continuum of responses from the health professionals with that of the patients to discover where there were significant differences in concerns and suggestions for action. We worked with these analyses to develop an interactive algorithm tool to assist health professionals to better meet the sexual and intimacy needs of people living with cancer.

Hordern, A. & Currow, D. 2003, 'A patient centred approach to sexuality in the face of life limiting illness', *The Medical Journal of Australia*, vol. 179, no. 6, pp. s8–s11.

Recommended reading

Berg, B.L. 2004, *Qualitative research methods for the social sciences*, Pearson, Boston.

Brannen, J. 1992, *Mixing methods: Qualitative and quantitative research*, Avebury, Aldershott.

Kellehear, A. 1993, *The unobtrusive researcher: A guide to methods*, Allen & Unwin, Sydney.

Rice, P.R. & Ezzy, D. 1999, *Qualitative research methods: A health focus*, Oxford University Press, Melbourne.

four

OBSERVATION AND PARTICIPANT OBSERVATION

Observation and participant observation, which involve observing people and situations in situ, are data collection methods with considerable benefits for health research. Unlike interviews or focus groups, observation and participant observation allow researchers to investigate social behaviour as it happens (Lofland & Lofland 1984). Qualitative researchers conducting observations rarely arrange their objects of study or change them, although they recognise that the very act of observation will have an effect and that any notes or records of the observation will reflect the viewpoint, background and knowledge of the observer. Consequently, where interviewing and focus groups can tell us what people have to say, observation and participant observation help us to see what actually happens.

What people say and what actually occurs can differ considerably (Lambert & McKevitt 2002; Rapp 1988). This has been demonstrated many times in studies where interview data and observation data are collected. One example concerns two studies of the eating habits of postpartum Malay women. When asked about their diet during interview, the participants stressed the importance of a restricted diet for postpartum women; however, observation showed that many of the women's diets varied considerably from their stated descriptions of an ideal postpartum diet (Laderman 1983; Wilson 1973). The opportunity to see what takes place in a particular setting rather than relying on participants' memories and interpretations allows researchers to address research problems that require knowledge of practice (Lambert & McKevitt 2002; Patton 1990:205).

Observation and participant observation also allow researchers to acquire background data about social settings or situations. This provides context for other types of data and may be used to identify key players who might be suitable for interviews or focus groups. It follows that they are useful methods to use at the beginning of a project where the researcher is trying to gain a feel for the research setting. For example, Cloherty et al. (2004) conducted research in a maternity unit in the south of England. They focused on the actions and beliefs of mothers and midwives towards supplemental bottle-feeding of breast-fed babies. Participant observation was used as the first stage in the data collection process. That data enabled the researchers to identify situations where supplemental feeding was offered as an option for mothers and to identify mothers and midwives to approach later for an interview.

Given the contrast between what people say and what occurs, it is no surprise that the ability to observe and participate in situations, settings, behaviours and actions often produces quite different findings to interview or focus group data. This is because many of the circumstances and factors that impact on what people do, why they do it that way, and how they feel about it are not 'always expressed orally, especially in one-off interviews which tend to produce orthodox responses' (Lambert & McKevitt 2002:211). Accordingly, perspectives gained through these methods may produce new interview or focus group questions (Caroleo 2001; Patton 1990:202).

Types of observation

There are two different ways to use observation as a data collection method in a qualitative research project. These are observing without participating and participant observation. In most studies where observation is used as a method, the researcher(s) will move between the two types of observation. Patton describes the extent of participation as a continuum with a great deal of variation (1990:206). The level of participation that is desirable or possible will vary according to the purpose of the research, the nature of the research setting and the characteristics of the researcher.

Observation

Simple observation involves systematically watching and sometimes also listening. A researcher using observation as a data collection tool is learning through watching and listening at a distance (Kellehear 1993).

An important aspect of this method is that the researcher avoids altering what they are observing any more than can be helped. Researchers observe details about the built environment, clothing, smells and sounds, repeated behaviours, body language and taken-for-granted actions. Observation can also help a researcher to see familiar situations in a markedly different way. It can jolt them out of everyday acceptance and allow for a sense of newness and strangeness.

Qualitative observation is a carefully planned activity, and researchers take detailed records called field notes. In a structured observation the researcher establishes clear guidelines for what behaviours are to be observed before they start the observation. Researchers may choose to focus on specific behaviours or actions or to focus on particular individuals. They generally use a checklist to record the frequency with which the specified behaviours are observed over a specified time. Researchers conducting a structured observation may also engage in 'priority observation' where they focus their observation on one person for a few minutes (recording speech, actions, appearance etc) and then shift their focus to another person for a few minutes, and so on (Carspecken 1996).

In contrast, in an unstructured observation, the researcher starts their recording with no pre-planned checklist of what will be observed. Instead they record behaviours, actions etc as they see them. Unstructured observation often becomes more structured over time as the researcher narrows down their area of interest. All observers should attempt to be active observers and to avoid lapses of concentration or 'daydreaming'. For this reason observation is extremely tiring and can only be practised for limited periods of time before the observer will need to rest (Clark & Bowling 1990).

Participant observation

Unlike observation without participation, participant observation involves experiencing events and situations from within. Instead of standing off to the side and observing from a distance, participant observation implies involvement, such as engaging in the activity being studied and talking with informants (Rice & Ezzy 1999:161). Some authors use the terms 'observer as participant' and 'partial observer' to give an indication of the level of participation. For example, a full participant observer is highly engaged in the activity or events. An 'observer as participant', or partial observer, is mainly engaged in observation but they may also speak with participants and engage in some aspects of the activity under study (Baker 1994:245).

Participant observation has a special advantage in that it allows researchers to understand a problem or situation through their own experience. Physically participating gives a vastly different perspective to simple observation or interviewing or conducting focus groups (Patton 1990:207). In a high-profile study of institutions, for example, Erving Goffman worked as an orderly in a mental institution (Goffman 1961). Participant observation as an employee gave him access to places, situations and experiences that would have been impossible if he had only visited the asylum as a guest conducting interviews. Participant observation data can also be collected by research participants and so provide an opportunity for their experiences to be analysed. For example, Chang et al. (2004) used participant observation data and reflective notes to supplement data from 15 interviewees in a study of the empowerment process for cancer patients. Participant observation data was collected by the interviewees and represented the experiences of the research participants.

Background to observation and participant observation

While observation and participant observation are methods used by researchers from a range of social scientific disciplines, they are most commonly associated with anthropological research. And, more specifically, with an anthropological methodology termed ethnography. Ethnographies are descriptive studies of cultures. Traditionally, ethnographies were conducted by anthropologists over a relatively long period of time and involved a researcher(s) living among the culture being studied, observing, participating and informally interviewing participants. Ethnographies aim to 'obtain and display in as much detail as possible, the understandings and meanings constructed by people as they undertake daily activities' (Grbich 1999:159). Participant observation and observation are methods also used in other types of field-based research. The term 'field work' arose during the early twentieth century when anthropologists and qualitative sociologists described themselves as working 'in the field' when they were collecting data. Fieldwork studies can be conducted from within a number of qualitative perspectives, including ethnography, phenomenology, grounded theory and case studies (Travers 2001).

A sub-field of anthropology known as medical anthropology has produced many ethnographic and fieldwork studies in medical settings (Guarnaccia 2001). While the majority of these are studies of non-Western cultures, medical anthropologists also use ethnographic methods such as observation and participant observation to investigate contemporary Western medicine. Examples include the training of medical specialists (Atkinson 1995), accident and emergency clinics (Dingwall & Murray 1983), fathers' participation in childbirth (de Carvalho 2003) and decision making by ear, nose and throat surgeons (Bloor 1976). Whittaker conducted an ethnographic study to explore community beliefs and practices concerning health and illness in an Australian town (Whittaker 1996).

There are also many notable examples of health-related ethnographies conducted by sociologists, public health researchers and nurse researchers (Leininger & McFarlane 2002; Leininger 1985). These are often smaller, more contained studies than the large-scale longitudinal ethnographies conducted in anthropology (Grbich 1999:158). Such studies usually combine observation and/or participant observation with interviews. For instance, observation and participant observation have been used in conjunction with interviews to allow public health researchers to learn about sexual and drug use practices (Power et al. 1996; Kotarba 1990). Ethnographic research is also used to inform the development of health-focused interventions, to investigate preventive behaviours such as solar protection behaviour among beachgoers (Devos et al. 2003) and to investigate the health of minority groups (Facey 2003).

The value of ethnography and field work lies in the level of detail and in-depth holistic understanding that such approaches achieve. This type of understanding encourages a 'cultural relativism, which is seeing the world from the people's own perspective' (Rice & Ezzy 1999:169). Ethnographic and other field-based research approaches lie at the heart of the qualitative research tradition.

Deciding to use observation or participant observation

Observation and participant observation offer researchers two different perspectives. As with other qualitative methods described in this book, deciding whether or not a method is suited to your research project requires careful consideration.

Observation is useful where the researcher requires:

1 Detailed information about context and settings.
2 To conduct unobtrusive research in public places.
3 Detailed field notes.

However, observation can only be conducted for relatively short periods of time on a relatively small number of people or places. It is also limited because the researcher is restricted to watching and listening. They are not supposed to interact with research participants. This can limit their capacity to understand the actions and events they are observing. These problems are largely overcome when using participant observation.

Participant observation is useful when the researcher requires:

1 To build rapport.
2 To engage with participants.
3 To break down distinctions between researcher and researched.
4 An insider perspective.

However, the interactive nature of participant observation means it can be a challenge to stay focused or take detailed notes. In addition, participant observation is often a complicated data collection method to organise. It can be difficult to obtain access to the field, and the ethical considerations can be complex (*see* Chapter Two). Participant observation is commonly used in studies where researchers are attempting to immerse themselves in a culture or situation (Zeitlyn & Rowshan 1997; Kaufert & O'Neill 1993). For example, a participant observation of general practice waiting rooms might entail attending waiting rooms as a patient or as the carer of a patient or working as a receptionist. It is also used in studies where the researcher is conducting research in a familiar setting in which they are already involved, such as their workplace, home or chronic illness support group. In these instances, it would be extremely difficult if not impossible to be a simple observer.

Being an observer

Textbooks about ethnography and field work often devote considerable space to discussions about the researcher's role (Berg 2004; Bailey 1996; Adler & Adler 1987). 'The position you assume or you are assigned to in the course of ethnographic research is referred to as a field role' (Marvasti 2004:50). As discussed in Chapter One, qualitative research demands a quite different researcher role to the objective and distanced role found in quantitative research. The researcher's role is relatively straightforward when conducting simple observation. However, when they move into participant observation, they find themselves in an interactive social situation with all of the associated complexities. The interactive nature of participant observation and the long periods of time that some participant observers spend with each research participant will inevitably produce changes in how a researcher views their role and their experiences in the field (Crick 1989). For example, when Julia Lawton conducted a participant observation study in a hospice (2001), she experienced role conflict. She found 'ambiguity inherent within an approach that requires a researcher to work simultaneously as a participant and as an observer' (Lawton 2001:693). Similarly, the case study example for this chapter was writtten by nurse researcher, Rosalind Bull. She conducted an observation in an operating theatre and found that the doctors and nurses working in that environment kept asking her to assist them by passing equipment etc.

Researchers are often advised to adopt roles that will be helpful to their field work. While it is not possible to change your age, sex or training, researchers do have flexibility in how they approach the research setting and other research participants. Lofland and Lofland (1984:15–16) describe two valuable stances, or roles, that researchers can adopt. They call the first of these the 'Martian'. Other writers have called this stance 'the stranger' (Schutz 1971). In this role, the researcher attempts to view a situation as an outsider with 'innocent' and 'fresh' eyes. The researcher considers their lack of knowledge to be an advantage because they hope it will allow them to notice 'taken-for-granted' behaviours and actions, and so on. A 'Martian' is likely to feel like an outsider and be treated as such by the research participants. It is equally possible that they will be looked after very well by the research participants, particularly if they are seen as eager to learn or 'charmingly incompetent'. The other stance is referred to as the 'convert'. The 'convert' hopes to gain understanding and insight by immersing themselves as completely as possible in the participants' ways of viewing the world. Adler and Adler (1987:64) call this type of field role 'active membership'. The deeper involvement associated with the 'convert' role may assist a researcher to gain greater insight. However, it also has implications for how they will feel about conducting the research. For example, they may start to feel disloyal or uncomfortable about writing and commenting on their 'friends'. Difficulties can also arise from a dislike or discomfort with the points of view of research participants (Rice & Ezzy 1999:170) An active field role also has the potential to change the researcher, as they become personally affected by the activities undertaken and the friendships made (Marvasti 2004:51). Some researchers are more successful than others in terms of their ability 'to experience other situations deeply, as if actually involved, to enter into the world of others and see their world from their viewpoint' (Baker 1994:238).

A common theme across discussions about a researcher's role in research projects involving observation and participant observation is the need for reflexivity and a critical self-awareness. Reflexivity requires insightfulness, receptivity and self-understanding (Baker 1994:238). Reflexive behaviours include reflecting about how your field role (or roles) might be impacting on the data collected and about how your own opinions, viewpoints and subject position might be impacting on the research. It is also important to reflect on how you are feeling about the research, the research participants and the project and record these reflections for later analysis (Finlay 2002:531–2). Participant observation is the method that most challenges traditional scientific distinctions between the researcher and the researched and notions that research requires distance and objectivity (Ellen 1984). The personal characteristics of the researcher, such as age, gender, social class, education and profession, will have a bearing on the ways that they *experience* behaviours or situations.

The important thing for new researchers to recognise is that fieldwork research will at times be emotional and that their role as a researcher is a complex one. Most researchers describe conducting field work as a mixed experience. Some describe feeling embarrassed, bored, lost or frightened while others describe excitement and satisfaction (Berg 2004:158; Perry 1989; Malinowski 1967). A researcher can experience all of these emotions in the one project.

Selecting research sites

Selecting appropriate places and groups of people to be the focus of an observation or participant observation requires great care. A well-selected site or group of research participants can improve the ease of running of the study and the quality of data obtained. Choosing places to conduct observation or participant observation and assessing their suitability and usefulness for the research project can happen in a number of different ways (Vallance 2001; Baker 1994).

How to select an observation site:

1 Be guided by the research problem and questions or by personal interests and concerns of the researcher.
2 Conduct a literature review to learn about suitable sites and groups.
3 Speak with possible participants or other knowledgeable individuals and ask their advice.

4 Chance encounters may lead to a research project and access to the field.
5 Take advantage of people, social networks and places familiar to you.
6 Forge research bargains to facilitate access (e.g. inviting a member of the group being studied to join the research team).

There are a number of issues to consider when choosing a research site. Researchers will need to think carefully about the characteristics of research participants and the nature of the research setting in relation to the research problem and questions. They should also consider the effect observation or participant observation might have on participants and the safety of the site or group for the researcher (Schatzman & Strauss 1973). Researchers may also need to consider their levels of knowledge about a particular setting or group and their capacity to become knowledgeable if they are not already (Baker 1994:242).

In some studies, lawfulness is a consideration; issues related to privacy, the risks of trespassing and of being present where illegal activity is underway come into play. Certain sites are obviously more risky than others; for example, public toilets, the headquarters of motorcycle gangs or criminal settings. However, the most common concern of qualitative researchers when selecting a research site is how easy it will be for them to gain entry to the site or group.

Some settings are more difficult than others to access. Variables include the nature of the settings, the purpose of the research and the identity of the researcher. For example, a young male student is likely to have more difficulties in accessing a breastfeeding support group than would a female. There may also be related issues about how much having a young male student in this group might inhibit the actions and discussions of the breastfeeding women. Sites such as prisons, elite settings, military settings and settings involving children are often particularly difficult to access unless the researcher has the support of someone inside the organisation or group (Hertz & Imber 1993; Spencer 1991).

In observation without participation, public spaces such as parks, sporting grounds and city streets may be suitable and these are usually easy to access. However, if the observation is to be conducted in a private space or within a setting such as a business, hospital, university or suchlike, then the researcher will need to obtain permission to conduct their observation. All participant observation will require either formal or informal permission. It is not uncommon for research questions to be altered once the researcher realises that they are unable to enter a suitable site (Rice & Ezzy 1999:170).

Gaining access

A great deal has been written about the difficulties associated with gaining access in field-based studies (Baker 1994:239; Lofland & Lofland 1984). Certainly having access is vital to the study: without access, no data can be gathered.

> Only after my arrival in the field did the problem of people's responses to the presence of a field worker occur to me. These responses, which in a large part were integral to the socio-cultural organisation of the community, produced an experience of field research for me that radically altered the initial focus of my project. Although I did not realise it at the time, my research was part of a social process that started from the very fact of my presence in the village. I had not anticipated the problems associated with explaining my presence in the village . . . (Mewett 1989:83)

A number of effective strategies has been developed for gaining access so the researcher can conduct their observation or participant observation. The first of these strategies is choosing a suitable site for your research. The next is strategic use of 'key informants' and 'gatekeepers' (Lofland & Lofland 1984:25). Key informants are knowledgeable individuals with connections to the research setting. Gatekeepers are individuals who, because of their role, have a great deal of influence. The most unlikely settings can be accessed if the researcher is assisted by key individuals (Berg 2004:159). For example, it is likely to be much more difficult to gain entry to a prison than to a community health centre for most researchers. However, if you have links with the prison through your work or the research project, then access may be achieved relatively simply. Similarly, a medically trained person is likely to find it much easier to go into certain medical settings than a layperson. Nonetheless, a layperson acquainted with a healthcare professional who works in the setting may find they are able to negotiate access.

After a researcher has gained access to a setting, they are likely to need to continually re-negotiate their level of access. For instance, as a researcher you may obtain permission to be in a particular location, but this does not ensure that the people working there will feel comfortable with your presence and agree to talk with you or allow you to participate. Winning their co-operation may take some time. Furthermore, because settings change, and the data needs of researchers shift, negotiating access tends to be an ongoing issue for researchers over the duration of their project (Lofland & Lofland 1984:20).

Recording data

After gaining access the next important issue is deciding how to record observations. Data are 'not the researcher's memories (which notes, interview write-ups, films and so forth merely assist); data consist of whatever is logged' (Lofland & Lofland 1984:47). So a study using observation and/or participant observation requires careful and focused data recording. These records are called field notes (Emerson et al. 1995:4). All records need to be carefully labelled with the time and location of the observation, the names or codenames for any research participants involved and any other important information of that nature (Chiseri-Strater & Sunstein 2001). It is helpful to prepare cover sheets for your notes with sections for this information. These can be stapled together at the end of the day.

In qualitative studies, researchers frequently begin their work by trying to become familiar with a setting or group of participants and take general notes. These might include notes about the setting, timeframes, the environment, people and their relationships, behaviour, actions and activities, verbal utterances and physical objects (Baker 1994). Later, as the study gets more refined, they may develop a more focused approach to their observation. A structured observation will require the use of an observation schedule.

Field notes

Field notes come in many different forms and may alter considerably over the course of a project (Fetterman 1989). If you are observing in order to get a feel for a situation or event, then your notes may be fairly informal and guided by the ebb and flow of events or whatever takes your interest. As your time spent observing grows, you will find that what you see changes, and this will be reflected in the style of your field notes (Burgess 1991:192; Bailey 1996:80–1). Berg (2004:174–5) describes the four distinct elements of field notes. Jottings are taken while in the field and may include sketches, unusual terms or phrases. They serve as a memory trigger. Detailed descriptions are 'the heart of any narrative field notes' (Berg 2004:174). The researcher writes these when they have left 'the field'. They should include as much detail as you can achieve. This includes describing the smells, sounds, actions and events observed. Analytic notes are ideas that occur to the esearcher while they are writing the field notes. For example, connections between observations and other aspects of the study, theories about what is happening or why, or questions about places, people and behaviours. Finally, subjective reflections are personal observations and comments about the researcher's feelings and experiences.

As an observer, it may be possible to take notes while you are observing. In some situations, however, you will need to withdraw after a period of observation and take notes in another location. Taking notes is more difficult for participant observers. Stopping to take notes would certainly constitute an interruption, and recording notes while actively engaging in an activity would make it difficult to participate. For this reason, participant observation is less suited to structured and detailed note taking.

Participant observers tend to withdraw and record notes at regular intervals or at the end of the day and use a combination of observation and participant observation. For example, Pranee Rice describes writing up field notes in her car after a session of participant observation and interviewing before she lost the sense of vividness and immediacy (Rice & Ezzy 1999:164). Bailey (1996:80–1) suggests that for participant observers, field notes can begin as 'mental notes' and brief jottings made when possible during the activity. These can assist with memory and recall when writing more detailed notes later in the day.

Observation also involves listening and possibly even asking questions, so your notes may need to record short informal interviews where you ask people for clarification or to explain what is happening. Having a micro cassette recorder or a digital recorder, as used by secretaries for taking transcription, can assist with easily recording these types of interview as well as your own observations. Remember, however, that talking into a recorder in front of people or while speaking with them could be extremely off-putting and distracting (Berg 2004:170). All audio notes should be transcribed and stapled together with any other written notes taken that day. Make copies and backups of your field notes and store these carefully. With the consent of participants, it is possible to videotape observations. This is useful as it allows a researcher to watch and review a particular setting or situation a number of times.

Observation schedules

Focused or structured observations frequently require an observation schedule. An observation schedule is a checklist of things to be recorded. They are often set out in a grid with sections to record time and location, specific activities, objects or other categories, plus the names or codenames of any research participants. Observation schedules are most useful for recording numerical data such as the number of people in a scene or the number of times a person performs a certain action or behaviour. The use of a schedule also allows for consistent record keeping, for large amounts of data to be recorded relatively quickly, and may improve inter-observer reliability.

Using observation and participant observation data

Observation and participant observation data lend themselves to a number of different uses. First, they can be the principal source of data for a research project. In such a case, field notes and any other data recorded would be analysed in much the same way as interview or focus group data. Second, they can be used in conjunction with other types of data, such as documents, interviews or focus groups. In these instances, the observation and participant observation data can be analysed independently, used by the researchers to assist in their analysis of the other types of data or to triangulate data (Fetterman 1989:89).

In my own work, I have found that even small amounts of observation and participant observation data can be valuable. They serve to prob-lematise other data by raising questions about any theories I might be developing about a situation or problem. Alternatively, they may raise new questions or strengthen a developing theory or hypothesis. Observation and participant observation data can give other data back-ground and context or simply be used to offer an alternative perspective that makes the research more interesting and rich. Conducting observation can also jolt a researcher into seeing familiar things in a new way, and keeping detailed observation notes and journal-type field entries is helpful in projects that span a long period of time. Re-reading them can take the researcher back and remind them of things that would be forgotten had they only used interview transcripts or focus group transcripts. For this reason, I recommend taking basic observation notes at the completion of interviews and focus groups, even in studies where observation data is not central to the overall project.

 Holstrom and Rosenqvist (2004) suggest an innovative way of using observation that may provide food for thought. They videotaped encounters between 18 patients with diabetes and their physician or diabetes nurse. These were transcribed and transcriptions given to the patients, who were then asked to reflect on the encounter. After this, each patient was interviewed. During the interview, the patient and the researcher watched the videotaped encounter and discussed issues such as the patient's views about the encounter, wider issues related to their healthcare and their understandings about diabetes. The interviews were then analysed.

Chapter summary

Observation and participant observation are data collection methods often used in ethnographic studies. However, both methods have advantages for most types of qualitative research design. Observation data provides the type of contextual background information that creates a rich and detailed qualitative study. The capacity for observation methods to allow a researcher to comment on practice is also invaluable. Participant observation is unique across the qualitative data collection methods because it permits a researcher to use their own experience as research data. It is also a highly flexible method allowing for informal interviewing and varying levels of researcher involvement. Further, it is a wonderful way to build rapport between researchers and research participants. Participant observation enables a researcher to build relationships with participants over a period of time. This has considerable benefits for the quality of data obtained, as is demonstrated in the following case study example from nursing researcher, Rosalind Bull.

Case study: Participant observation in the operating theatre: 'Theatre wear must be worn beyond this point'

Dr Rosalind Bull, Senior Lecturer in Nursing, University of Tasmania, Australia

The success of any fieldwork endeavour depends inherently on the results of the unofficial study the observed undertake of the observer (Van Maanen 1988:31).

Research that seeks to create understanding about the way in which nurses, the people for whom they care and the environment interact tends to be best achieved using a qualitative rather than quantitative design. Unlike quantitative work, qualitative research allows the researcher to examine multiple interpretations of the truth, thus capturing the complexity of the nursing experience. The practice of nursing, and therefore much of the related research, is holistic. For example, nursing acknowledges the importance of social and cultural dimensions to health, as well as the biophysical aspects. To this end nurses accept that people and the way in which they perceive the truth about their world is an individual interpretation.

In my project, I wanted to capture the contribution of nurses to the work of the operating room. I wanted to know what they did, when they did it, how they did it, who they did it with and why they did it. From this I then wanted to be able to analyse my findings in terms of the culture of the operating room. Ethnography provided me with the best methods to gather the data needed to answer my questions. To undertake a study using ethno-graphic methods I needed to undertake a substantial amount of fieldwork in the operating room (OR) itself.

There is a shortage of new nurses in OR nursing. The average age of OR nurses is increasing. Nursing students receive limited exposure to the OR and tend not to choose OR nursing as a preferred career option on graduation. Technicians and other auxiliary workers are beginning to take over traditional nursing activities in the area, and policy makers are very keen on this cheaper and readily available alternative. And then there's the place itself. The OR is isolated from the busy world of the hospital, its staff wear a different uniform, they work by different rules and they do different things. Looking through the theatre doors is like looking into a different world. And it is. The OR is a culture all of its own.

The operating room above all is an uncompromisingly technological space. Its physical landscape is minimalist and functional, which is a direct reflection of its main purpose – the conduct of surgical procedures by surgeons. The patients are anaesthetised or sedated depending on the pro-cedure and are almost completely submerged under layers of sterile green drapes. So why, when it is so obviously a technical area, would you have nurses in there? This question has dogged the OR nursing profession. Explicit and exacting justification for the presence of nurses in the technological world of the OR is hard to come by. Intuitively it makes sense to have nurses, with their patient focus and attendant ethics present where the most vulner-able of all patients are, but policy makers demand more than intuition. My research entitled 'Theatre wear must be worn beyond this point' sought to cast light on the contribution that nurses make to the work of the OR.

Fieldwork is the central activity of all ethnographers and is done to study life as it is lived. Participant observation is one of the principal methods used to conduct fieldwork. For research that examines human activity within a cultural framework, participant observation offers a vehicle to gather infor-mation on such things as the way in which the people within a particular culture act, how they relate to each other, how time, space and objects are used. In other words, it enables researchers to gather information that answers questions like: What? How? When? Who and who with? (thereby having the additional merit of appealing to the gossip in all of us). In my study fieldwork helped me to gain some understanding of the OR culture render-ing the hidden and taken-for-granted things of this unique culture visible and thereby examinable.

The study used participant observation as one of the main fieldwork methods. I made just over 220 hours of observations in 71 visits. During that time I developed hundreds of pages of field notes using three stages of field noting. In the first stage, done during and shortly after observation, I made brief handwritten preliminary notes on what I had observed. I then expanded these into comprehensive, concrete descriptions that could be analysed. These expanded field notes were then annotated with interpretations, comments, cross references and links with the literature and thus became the analytical field notes.

During the data collection phase of my study I found that theory only went so far in helping me develop as a participant observer. Making the preliminary notes, for example, proved to be an unexpected challenge. The books that I had read advised me to take notes immediately and I dutifully took my notebook into the theatre. I soon found that each time I made a note people would stop what they were doing to have a look at what I had just written. This disrupted the observation (not to say the operation) so I had to tailor my observation periods to allow me to leave the room and make notes. I had also underestimated the difficulty I would have in hearing what people were saying through their surgical masks. I compounded this problem by initially adhering to theory that observations should be done from an unobtrusive position, but sadly I chose to stand in a corner near the CD player which was off at the time. Once the operation had started, however, the steady strains of new-age country & western made it impossible for me to hear anything at all.

Access was another issue where flexibility was demanded. To conduct the observations I had to gain access to the OR and having jumped the formal and informal hoops presented by ethics clearance, permission from the Director of Nursing, managers and staff I had thought myself to free to observe. To my surprise I found that my access to the study setting was fragile and fluctuated constantly. The intensity of my observation of the nurses was matched by their observation of me. Was I safe to be in the theatre? Was I really observing what I said I would observe? Was I evaluating their nursing care? Could I be trusted?

One-to-one conversation, work-in-progress meetings and making my field notes accessible to the nurses helped gain trust on one level. I found that active concentration on acceptable behaviour within the OR environment prevented me blundering through cultural rules to some extent but some of the rules were hidden and had to be learnt by trial and error. For example, I learnt the 'avoid touching anything green' rule very quickly but took a longer time working out that the circulating nurse rather than the instrument nurse should be my first port of call on entering the theatre.

My main role in the fieldwork was 'observer as participant'. This role placed the emphasis firmly on observation (the principal object), but meant that I had the flexibility to participate in ways that assisted the maintenance of access. Combining a minimal level of clinical participation with a high level of observation also emphasised the research side of my relationship with the nurses and de-emphasised our clinical relationship. I found that striking a balance between observer and participant roles involved more than a reiteration of the purpose of observation, it meant clearly defining what role I was playing at the time. The roles of clinician, friend and researcher were all interwoven throughout the fieldwork and each of the roles was important to its success. My role as researcher was central, the other two roles, while at times confusing the issue, contributed to gaining and maintaining access and collecting the rich in-depth data for the study.

So what have been the outcomes thus far from this study? I have had three publications in international journals and have spoken at several conferences as well as to interested groups of OR nurses. The need to publish and get the work out there cannot be over-stressed. There have been a few very pleasing changes that have occurred as a result of the study. In one instance, an OR manager (a non-nurse) is now aware of what the nurses call 'surgeon's time'. That is the amount of time the surgeon believes an operation will take (often an underestimate) as opposed to the amount of time it will really take. This manager now includes the nurses as well as the surgeons in the theatre scheduling and as a result, stress related to overly tight schedules has been reduced. In another department the study has been used to manage some difficult staff behaviour. As far as influencing policy goes, the findings have been included in information being gathered as part of a current inquiry into OR nursing. On a personal level the study was challenging and tremendously satisfying. I gained a new and refreshing perspective on an area of nursing practice about which I knew very little. Doing the study has helped me to become more observant, more open-minded to different interpretations and more rigorous in the way I think about research.

Van Maanen, J. 1988, *Tales of the field: On writing ethnography*, University of Chicago Press, Chicago.

Recommended reading

Bailey, C.A. 1996, *A guide to field research*, Pine Forge Press, Thousand Oaks.

Hammersley, M. & Atkinson, P. 1995, *Ethnography: Principles in practice*, 2nd edn, Routledge, New York.

Lofland, J. & Lofland, L. 1984, *Analyzing social settings: A guide to qualitative observation and analysis*, 2nd edn, Wadsworth, Belmont.

Malinowski, B. 1967, *A diary in the strict sense of the term*, Routledge, London.

Perry, J. 1989, *Doing fieldwork: Eight personal accounts of social research*, Deakin University Press, Geelong.

five
INTERVIEWING

Interviews collect information about the ways that people understand 'the events and experiences of their lives' (Grbich 1999:85). They are a flexible way of collecting qualitative data suited to a wide variety of projects and research methodologies. For example, interviews have been used to explore a range of health-related issues, including the preferences of terminal cancer patients regarding their place of death (Thomas et al. 2004), young women's views on the relationship between cigarette smoking and weight control (Nichter et al. 2004), male narratives of pregnancy loss (McCreigh 2004), and how people manage living with a chronic illness (Charmaz 1990 and 1991).

Unlike observation and participant observation, interviews produce 'second-order data' because interviews involve discussion of events or experiences that have already occurred (Grbich 1999:86). Interviews can be used as the only method of data collection in a project or in combination with other methods.

There are at least four distinct styles of interviewing. These are structured interviews, semi-structured interviews, unstructured in-depth interviews and short informal interviews. Interviews can be conducted person-to-person and using telephones. Recent technological advances have made it possible to conduct interviews on-line, using email and via video-link. They can also be conducted between two people (an interviewer and an interviewee) or in a group (most commonly one interviewer and two or more interviewees). This chapter focuses exclusively on person-to-person interviews conducted with no more than three people because this is the type of interviewing most routinely used in health-related qualitative research.

The chapter begins with a short discussion about the history of interviewing as a data collection method. It then describes in some detail three types of interview – in-depth, semi-structured and structured interviews. The chapter also provides practical guidance related to conducting interviews and collecting interview data. It closes with a case study from an experienced qualitative interviewer, Jon Adams, Director, Qualitative Research Laboratory at a regional university. His case study describes a research project investigating the views of general practitioners about complementary and alternative medicine.

Background to interviewing

Interviews are used in fields as diverse as journalism, education and medicine and in situations such as television shows, radio, recruitment, the courts and in law enforcement. Atkinson and Silverman have stated that because of the widespread use of interviews across such a broad range of fields and situations, interviewing is now seen as a natural mode of gathering information (Atkinson & Silverman 1997).

As with other data collection methods, the ways in which interviews are conducted varies considerably depending on a project's methodology and the purpose of the research. However, in the main, qualitative interviews conducted for purposes of research are quite different to other types of interview in common use (Gubrium & Holstein 2002). In qualitative research, interviewers are particularly interested in eliciting the views of the interviewee and so tend to avoid the use of controlling interview styles or structured interview questions, choosing instead more relaxed and conversational styles of interviewing that facilitate in-depth understanding and reciprocity of exchange (Warren et al. 2003).

Interviewing has waxed and waned in popularity among social researchers. Fontana and Frey (2003:66–8) describe largely informal qualitative interviewing combined with field work and observation as a popular method in the Chicago School (a type of sociology practised in North America in the 1920s and '30s). However, qualitative interviewing was later largely submerged as a data collection method in the 1940s and '50s by the increasing popularity of survey research and standardised interviewing. Semi-structured interviewing was then developed as a distinct method in the 1960s. It was closely associated with empirically focused sociological perspectives, such as symbolic interactionism, ethnomethodology and phenomenology, and researchers such as Erving Goffman, Alfred Schutz, and Norman Denzin (Mischler 1979, 1986; Denzin 1970; Schutz 1967). These interviews were conducted in a relatively standardised fashion, and considerable attention was paid to rigorous methods and technique. However, the majority of social scientific research utilised quantitative methods, such as surveys and questionnaires (Fontana & Frey 2003:67). Similarly, while interviewing has always been a core data collection method in anthropology, these have tended to be short, relatively informal interviews conducted as part of participant observation or in a largely standardised manner.

Qualitative interviewing as a distinct data collection method re-emerged in the 1970s and '80s alongside the increasing popularity of naturalistic qualitative research (Lofland & Lofland 1984). Seidman (1998) stresses that the development of this type of interviewing parallels the development of contemporary qualitative research because in-depth and largely unstructured interviews are an acknowledgment that the 'subjects of inquiry in the social sciences can talk and think . . . at the very heart of what it means to be human is the ability of people to symbolize their experience through language' (1998:2). It follows that while methods such as observation or surveying enable researchers to observe and quantify behaviours and actions, open-ended and relatively unstruc-tured qualitative interviewing allows a researcher to explore how people view their own behaviours and experiences, and the meanings they attribute to them.

Interviewing is a popular method in health-related research (Rice & Ezzy 1999:65). It is a data collection method closely associated with the types of methodology – for example, grounded theory, phenomenology and ethnography – frequently used in fields such as nursing, primary care and public health research (Lopez & Willis 2004; Guarnaccia 2001). Interviews are also a standard method in health-related qualitative research conducted by sociologists and medical anthropologists. They are popular because they allow researchers to investigate issues from the perspectives of those involved. This could include decision-making processes; beliefs about health, illness and medical practices; and the meanings given to events or actions (Cornford et al. 2004; Donner 2003; Daly et al. 1992). While interviews alone cannot provide the depth of understanding achievable through participant observation, they allow for far greater detail than focus groups. For example, Low et al. (2004) used interviews to explore the impact of domiciliary and day hospital delivery of stroke rehabilitation on informal carers.

When contemporary health-related interview studies are examined, a tension is apparent between traditional social science research interviews and a more recent understanding of interviews arising from postmodern, feminist and narrative theory (Marvasti 2004:31). The traditional interview is based on three assumptions (Gubrium & Holstein 2002). First, that human beings share a common experience. Consequently, researchers assume that each person's opinions and views are valid and that interviewing an appropriate selection of people will give the researcher insight with a broader applicability (Marvasti 2004:15). Second, that in the majority of instances, the interviewer and the interviewee (respondent or informant) will adopt two recognised and active roles. The interviewer role is akin to that of a leader and the interviewee's role, a follower. 'The rhythmic give-and-take of this exchange is something that most of us are familiar with and take for granted' (Marvasti 2004:16). The third assumption underpinning traditional research interviews is that interview respondents are seen as a source of answers or 'vessels of answers' responding to the interviewer's questioning (Gubrium & Holstein 1997:119). Accordingly, it is assumed that if the interviewer asks the 'right questions' they will receive the answers they require. From this perspective, interviews are seen as a tool to gain insight into the ways that people make sense of the world or the things that they do, a way of 'finding out' what is going on.

Contrasting understandings of interviewing emerged in the 1980s and '90s from postmodernism, narrative theory, discourse analysis and some feminist and literary theories (Fontana & Frey 2003:67; Mischler 1986; Oakley 1981). From these alternative perspectives, interviews are seen as a creative and interactive process whereby the interviewer and the interviewee participate in a joint construction of events and interpretations (Denzin 1989). A well-known version of this new way of conceptualising interviewing is Holstein and Gubrium's (1997) description of the 'active interview'. Active interviewing entails awareness about 'how meaning and reality are created through interactions that are embedded in the social occasion of the interview' (Marvasti 2004:30). It follows that: 'All participants in an interview are inevitably implicated in making meaning' (Holstein and Gubrium 1997:126). From this understanding, interviewees are no longer viewed as a 'vessel of answers' and interviewers as a source of questions. Rather interviews are seen as 'speech events in which meanings are negotiated and reformulated' (Rice & Ezzy 1999:53). Interviews are social occasions in their own right 'whereby researchers and respondents jointly create social reality through interaction' (Marvasti 2004:29).

The impact of this newer perspective on interviewing is evident in recent interview studies (Seidman 1998; Roulston et al. 2003). Common themes are researcher reflexivity, recognition of the interactive and contextual nature of interviews and a concern about the 'ownership' of stories that emerge during interviews. Marvasti (2004:30) describes active interviewing as being 'less about how-to technical procedures than as a way of conceptualising and analyzing the interview process'.

Types of interview

At least four different types of interviewing are described in the qualitative research literature. These are standardised interviews, semi-structured interviews, in-depth unstructured interviews and informal interviews. Each of these is associated with certain methodological perspectives. However, in addition to methodology, deciding on the most appropriate type of interviewing for a project is closely linked with the issue being investigated, the social context for the research, the character-istics of the research participants and the style and attributes of the researcher. Different styles of interviewing tend to suit different research purposes. Grbich suggests that researchers should trial different types of interviewing during a preliminary or 'pilot' stage in their research project to assist them in choosing the most useful style for their particular project (1999:84). This advice is also given by Seidman, who states, 'I urge all interviewing researchers to build into their proposal a pilot venture in which they try out their interviewing design with a small number of participants' (1998:32). It is important to note, however, that 'pilots' are a contested issue in qualitative research. It is difficult to quarantine a set of interviews as a 'pilot' phase in inductive research designs where all data can be seen as part of the overall study. Researchers conducting trial interviews will need to decide how this data is to be used and potentially view all of their interviews as part of the overall project rather than as 'pilot' and 'non-pilot' interviews.

Structured interviews

Structured interviews aim to collect data that is readily coded and quanti-fied. Interviewers use a list of questions with a limited choice of closed response categories. This allows them to record answers according to a pre-established coding scheme (Fontana & Frey 2003:68). When conducting structured interviews, an interviewer attempts to replicate the same interview each time with a new interviewee. To assist with this, interviewers receive training in how to ask the question, how to minimise interaction with the interviewee and how to respond to any questions they are asked about the study.

This style of interviewing is an attempt to minimise bias or subjectiv-ity; it is clearly derived from positivist research where objectivity is an aim (Blaikie 1993). As such, structured interviews are not readily classi-fiable as a qualitative research method. They are best suited to situations where researchers want similar information to that obtainable through a questionnaire. Structured interviewing has advantages in situations where respondents are unable to complete a questionnaire. The addition of open-ended questions will also allow for qualitative data to be collected (Grbich & Sykes 1989). Grbich (1999:94) suggests that structured open-ended interviews are useful if a researcher wants to collect qualitative data from a large number of participants and to compare the data.

Nevertheless, structured interviews 'often elicit rational responses, but overlook or inadequately assess the emotional dimension' (Fontana & Frey 2003:70). In addition, structured interviews are based on a number of assumptions largely incompatible with qualitative research. They assume that 'it is possible to structure and order all questions in a manner that ensures they have the same meaning for all participants' (Denzin 1989:104). They assume that it is possible to avoid bias or to replicate an interactive event such as an interview. And that there is 'only one correct answer or version of events' (Rice & Ezzy 1999:54).

Semi-structured interviews

In semi-structured interviews, also called focused interviews, the interviewer uses a list of interview questions (an interview guide); however, these questions are open-ended. Furthermore, the interviewer is not bound by any expectations that they will ask the same questions at each interview, nor that they will ask them in the same way – unlike structured open-ended interviewing. Instead, the interview guide is there to help the interviewer to remember topics they want included in the interview. Interviewers are also free to ask additional questions during the interview and to respond to issues or questions raised by the interviewee.

Semi-structured interviews are closely associated with inductive methodologies, such as grounded theory. Interview guides are dynamic because they reflect ongoing data collection and analysis. It often happens that the questions or topics in one interview are those raised in earlier interviews or ones which have emerged from a preliminary analysis as being interesting and relevant. However, it is also assumed that an interviewer cannot know all relevant questions before they start the interview (Rice & Ezzy 1999:54). Accordingly, they are expected to ask additional questions to clarify answers given by the interviewee and to follow new lines of questioning if these emerge during the interview. Researchers using semi-structured interviews are likely to interview a research partici-pant several times, building on earlier interviews and asking new questions developed after interviewing other research participants (Hansen 2001). Conducting several interviews also provides an opportunity for research participants to reflect on their earlier interviews and the issues being discussed. Seidman strongly recommends this technique, arguing that 'interviewers who propose to explore their topic by arranging a one-shot meeting with an "interviewee" whom they have never met tread on thin contextual ice' (1998:11).

Semi-structured interviewing draws on very different skills to those of structured interviewing. Interviewers need to build rapport, listen carefully and allow pauses and thinking time for the research participant. Unlike structured interviews, it is also appropriate – and often necessary – for the interviewer to respond to the interviewee; for example, by showing interest, curiosity, a sense of humour and, in some cases, emotional support (Rice & Ezzy 1999:57). However, it should always be remembered that your role as an interviewer in a semi-structured interview is to provide a space for the interviewee to elaborate on their views and experiences related to the issue of inquiry. When transcripts from these types of interview are examined, the interviewer should be seen to speak considerably less often than the interviewee.

Semi-structured interviews are less predictable than structured interviews. They tend to vary in length and can be hard work for the interviewer (Seidman 1998:26). Remembering questions and thinking of new questions while at the same time trying to conduct a 'naturally' flowing conversation and listen carefully to the interviewee is a bit like juggling. Furthermore, because semi-structured interviews represent a halfway point between the objective standardised interview and unstructured in-depth interviews, they carry a range of often-competing expectations. On one hand, semi-structured interviews require to some degree the maintenance of traditional interviewer/interviewee roles. The interviewer has a set of issues or topics to discuss and they attempt to keep the conversation focused around these. On the other hand, interviewers are expected to build rapport and to give of themselves instead of remaining a neutral and distant figure. They should also avoid being controlling or dominant, instead allowing the conversation and levels of disclosure to be driven by the interviewee.

Unstructured in-depth interviews

Unstructured in-depth interviews are characterised by a largely informal approach and are marked by a lack of distance between the interviewer and interviewee (Mischler 1986). 'Unstructured interviews are shared experiences in which researchers and interviewees come together to create a context of conversational intimacy in which participants feel comfortable telling their story' (Corbin & Morse 2003:338). This style of interviewing emphasises the expertise of the interviewee, in contrast to structured interviewing, where the power lies with the interviewer (Marcus & Fischer 1986).

In-depth unstructured interviewing is a method stemming from perspectives such as phenomenology and narrative theory, where researchers want to understand the meanings people give to their experiences, to study the stories they tell and to place these in context. Therefore, the purpose of in-depth interviews is not to get answers to questions to evaluate or test hypotheses. Instead in-depth interviews reflect an interest in understanding other people's experiences and the meanings they attribute to those experiences.

A basic assumption in in-depth interviewing research is that the meaning people give to their experiences affects the way they carry out that experience. To observe a teacher, student, principal or counsellor, for example, provides access to their behaviour only. Interviewing allows us to put behaviour in context and provides access to understanding their actions (Seidman 1998:4).

While these types of interview are described as unstructured because they rarely make use of pre-established interview questions, the researcher is still acutely aware of the issues or topics they are interested in pursuing. The researcher conducting the interview will often ask the interviewee to clarify or expand on issues and will ask questions related to the interview topic. However, this is often done after they have concluded their narrative for fear of intruding on the narrative process (Corbin & Morse 2003:339). In order to build rapport and trust, interviewers conducting unstructured in-depth interviews may tell the interviewee about themselves and how they came to be conducting the research. This includes describing any personal connections with the topic under study (Grbich 1999:98; Thompson 1995).

Researchers such as Seidman (1998) and Rosenthal (2003) describe the large amounts of preparation and planning necessary before an unstructured interview. For example, Seidman (1998) suggests that researchers should plan to hold three interviews with each research participant. The first interview provides the research participant with an opportunity to tell the interviewer as much as possible about themselves in light of the topic under investigation (1998:11). This often involves discussing life history, early experiences and placing the issue under investigation in a context. The purpose of the second interview is to 'concentrate on details of the participant's present experience in the topic area of study' (1998:12). The third interview builds on the two earlier interviews. It provides an opportunity for reflection on meaning and making 'intellectual and emotional connections' (1998:12).

Unstructured and in-depth interviews have produced numerous important findings in health-related research (Morse 1989; Mischler 1986). They also facilitate many of the ideals of contemporary qualitative

research, among them reflexivity and minimising differential power relationships between researchers and research participants. The intimacy
and trust associated with this type of interviewing is the complete
opposite of the distance and control valued in quantitative research
methods (Corbin & Morse 2003:338).

However, this style of interviewing has been criticised for assuming
that experience equates with authenticity and is somehow more important or 'real' (Atkinson & Silverman 1997; Silverman 1997). It is also
difficult to reconcile the informal and intimate nature of this type of
interviewing with the bureaucratic requirements of most health-related
research projects; for example, informed consent forms, submitting interview questions to ethics committees or funding bodies, and expectations
about the ownership of intellectual property acquired during the course
of research. Combining the roles of unstructured in-depth interviewer
and scholar (or evaluator) is likely to be difficult at times (Fontana &
Frey 2003:96). Despite this, the benefits can be considerable.

Informal interviews

Informal interviews are brief interviews held as an opportunity arises
(Heyl 2001). They often occur during participant observation. Spradley
(1979) describes these types of interview as friendly conversations.
Interview questions are usually spontaneous and are 'based on interaction
between the researcher and the respondent' (Grbich 1999:93). Informal
interviews may also occur before or after a formal interview. These interviews are often recorded in field notes and can be highly valuable. Grbich
suggests that these types of interview can serve as a useful starting point
for formal interviews (1999:93).

Being an interviewer

Interviewers face concerns similar to those described in the previous
chapter on observation and participant observation. They need to access a
setting, understand the language and culture of the research participants,
decide how to present themselves, and gain trust and build rapport
(Fontana & Frey 2003). As you can see from this list, interviewers are the
data collection tool and so their attributes, personal characteristics, knowledge and life experience will impact on the interviews they conduct. This
includes how they think about the world, how they make sense of those
around them, and how others will view them (Roulston et al. 2003:650).
For example, a study investigating the impact of an interviewer's

professional role on interaction in in-depth interviews found that being seen as a 'doctor' or alternatively as a 'young woman' impacted on interaction during in-depth interviews (Richards & Emslie 2000). For this reason, it is important to spend some time reflecting on the advantages and limitations associated with your being who you are or how you might appear (Fine & Weis 1998).

Consider the impression you want to convey with your appearance and any written or telephone communication with the interviewees. Once 'the interviewers presentational self is "cast", it leaves a profound impression on the respondents and has a great influence over the success (or lack of it) of the study' (Fontana & Frey 2003:77). As a general rule, I think it best to seem friendly, of good intent and lowly in status. Hermanowitcz describes this as 'playing the innocent' or appealing to the research participant's altruism (2002:486).

However, interviewing elites such as doctors, lawyers or politicians may provide an exception to this (Meredith 1993; Daly & McDonald 1992; Fox 1992). When interviewing elites, an interviewer may need to convince them of their competency. For example, when I was a PhD student interviewing medical practitioners, I found that some of them were reluctant to engage with me until I began using medical terminology and revealed knowledge about certain epidemiological texts and authors. After this they began to engage in discussion (Hansen 2001).

Another important issue associated with conducting interviews is language. This refers to the language used by the interviewer, the language used by the interviewee and the capacity of each to understand the other. The literature is full of examples of researchers having problems communicating with the people they are interviewing because of language issues (Hammersley & Atkinson 1995). These difficulties vary from interviewers and interviewees speaking completely different languages to subtle differences of meaning among speakers of the same language (Harris & Roberts 2003; Wax 1960). Within any society or group of same-language speakers, there are variations in language usage that reflect gender, class and other differences (Dunbar et al. 2002; Kong et al. 2002). As researchers in health, you will be familiar with the difficulties of communication that arise between those with medical training and those without, and sometimes between those with different types of medical training.

For these reasons, no researchers using interviewing as a data collection method can afford to ignore issues of language. You will need to think about how to best facilitate effective interviews. Are you the best person to conduct the interviews? Perhaps the interviews should be prefaced with a period of observation and exploration during which you familiarise yourself with the individuals or group you are interested in? Is the most effective approach for you to interview as a naïve beginner openly questioning the meanings of various terms or would it be more useful to demonstrate knowledge and gain rapport that way? If you are using the services of a translator, what impact is this likely to have on the interviews?

Another issue is how an interviewer conducts themself while in the field. To a large degree this was addressed in Chapters Two and Three in relation to research ethics. As stated there, a researcher should be professional, respectful and always considerate towards research participants. However, semi-structured and unstructured interviews require an interviewer to spend time with research participants in an informal and relaxed manner. This can throw up new challenges, as interviewers have to use their everyday social skills. It is important not to rush through the beginning stages of an interview or the final stages after the interview has been completed. Both of these stages should be handled carefully, and an interviewer should be guided by the behaviour and conduct of the interviewee (Warren et al. 2003; Morse & Field 1995:98).

The final topic in this section is interviewing vulnerable or marginalised people or conducting interviews dealing with sensitive or emotional topics. These might include interviews with young people or the aged, refugees, disabled people or people living with an illness. These types of interview require the interviewer to be particularly careful and sensitive to the needs of the interviewee. They are also highly dependent on the skills of the interviewer. Harris and Roberts (2003) advise interviewers to identify anything that may impact on an interviewee's capacity to participate in an interview and plan how these barriers will be overcome. They suggest that a flexible and inventive approach should enable interviewers to conduct these types of interview. They also recommend that researchers provide more time in their research timetable and factor in additional costs (2003:15). Corbin and Morse (2003), writing about interviews dealing with sensitive topics, argue that when interviews are 'conducted with sensitivity and guided by ethics' they can be productive and beneficial for both parties.

Planning the interview

Planning an interview is in some ways similar to planning a participant observation. Initially, a researcher needs to identify suitable people to interview, recruit them to the study and schedule appointments. Decisions about sampling are discussed in Chapter Three. Identifying interviewees is often a fluid process. For example, it might be clear in your research plan that you aim to interview 40 nurses with a range of different levels of experience in aged-care nursing. However, actually finding these nurses will probably involve a number of different strategies. Examples include advertising, contacting aged care facilities or hospitals, approaching professional organisations, making use of contacts and asking for suggestions from nurses you have already interviewed. Recruitment for interviews is often a challenge. It always takes longer than you expect and it is helpful to use a number of different methods. The most important lessons I have learnt are to follow up interested people as quickly as possible and to locate key informants and ask them to help recruit potential interviewees.

Location

The next step in planning an interview is to select suitable locations. It is usual in qualitative interviewing to allow the research participants to choose the location for their interview. Many interviews will occur in homes, workplaces or public venues (Rice & Ezzy 1999:62; Taylor & Bogdan 1998). However, in health-related research projects, the research is often conducted in medical settings; for example, in hospital wards or clinics. While this is often convenient, it may generate problems, such as interview participants feeling vulnerable or health practitioner researchers falling back onto the case history and adopting interview styles commonly used during a consultation. These potential problems can be overcome if the interviewer is aware of them.

The key features to look for in an interview location are that it feels safe and comfortable, it is relatively quiet and undisturbed, and that it is accessible. My first sociology professor told my class that when conducting an interview in a participant's home, the best place to hold the interview is at the kitchen table. Kitchens are usually comfortable, informal and warm. The table provides a great place for two people to sit closely to each other while still feeling protected. They also make it easy to lean in towards each other and to sit the tape recorder at an appropriate height. He stressed the importance of sitting at a table corner so that you and the interviewee are at an angle, rather than sitting opposite each other. Many participants will want to sit in the 'best room' or in lounge chairs. However, I often request the kitchen or at least a table. When sitting in lounge chairs, the interviewee is often too far away from the interviewer. This makes it difficult to place a tape recorder where it will capture both voices, and the participant will often get up to fetch something or to move around the room, putting themselves out of range of the tape recorder.

It is important to try and find a quiet space where interruptions can be minimised. This can be impossible if people have little children or pets (Roulston et al. 2003). One of my recent interviews is unintelligible on the tape because of the constant barking of a dog. Eventually, the interviewee let the dog into the room, then it climbed all over us and wanted to lick my face. Although this was bad for our concentration and focus, it certainly broke the ice.

If you have chosen semi-structured or unstructured interviewing, some interruptions can be useful. For example, I once arrived for an interview with an elderly man and found that his wife was also waiting to speak with me. Initially, I was concerned because I had not planned to conduct a group interview. However, in this case it proved to be an asset because she seemed to spur him on to talk and she challenged him on some points. Since this experience, I often ask elderly male interviewees if they would like their partner to be part of the interview.

What to take with you

I have recently realised that travelling to an interview is a little bit like travelling with a young child. It doesn't pay to travel light. The following items are all necessary: recording gear, information about the study, any information you have about the participant (e.g. phone number, address), ethics forms, street directory, notebook and pen. In some studies it is also appropriate to take a small gift. It is useful to take a mobile phone – remember to turn it off before you begin the interview. This has two purposes. If you arrive for the interview and the participant is nowhere to be found, you can phone them. Mobile phones are also a useful safety backup for the interviewer in case something unexpected happens, such as a car breakdown.

Interviewer and interviewee safety is an important issue to consider. An interviewer should always tell someone where he or she is going and roughly how long he or she expects to be. In some studies when I was conducting interviews in a research participant's home, I chose to have a partner wait for me in the car. If the interview topic is likely to pose safety problems for the interviewee – for example, in interviews focused on abortion, drug use or criminal activity – it may be safer to conduct the interviews in an anonymous location so that no one can identify the interviewee as being associated with the activity.

Before the interview

There are several important steps to follow before starting an interview (Morse & Field 1995:98). When an interviewer (or interviewee) arrives for an interview, it is usual to begin with greetings, offers of tea or coffee and a generalised discussion about the project. The interviewer and the interviewee may feel nervous and need time to settle in and get to know each other. Many researchers take this opportunity to explain their interest in the research problem and to tell the interviewee about themselves (Rice 1996; Grbich 1999). The interviewer then needs to read over with the research participant any vital information about the project and the interview. They may need to answer questions about how the interview data will be recorded and used by the researcher, and explain how confidentiality will be maintained. It is important to take this opportunity to ask the interviewee if they are happy for the interview to be recorded and to explain if any written notes will also be taken (Roulston et al. 2003:650). After this, informed consent forms usually need to be signed.

After the interview

Warren et al. (2003) describe a distinct strip of time between the end of an interview and leave-taking. In some projects this strip of time is quite brief. Both the interviewer and the interviewee are happy to take their leave (DeSantis 1980). An interview can be quite a tiring experience and it will often come to a fairly natural end for both parties (Hermanowicz 2004:487). Nevertheless, in some instances interviewees are reluctant to stop the interview. They may be lonely, socially isolated or just enjoying the experience of reflecting on their lives (Marvasti 2004; Wenger 2001; Humphreys 1970). In these cases, the interviewer may be asked to stay and dine or to continue talking. How a researcher responds to this is personal. Some researchers are happy to engage in this type of socialising with research participants. Others consider it is inappropriate and may feel uncomfortable.

The degree of follow-up for research participants varies from study to study. Most ethics committees require the researcher to provide research participants with their contact details so that they can contact the researcher with any questions or concerns. It is worth reflecting about how you plan to provide follow-up for your research participants. The easiest way to manage this is to ask your participants if they would like to be followed up. Some will not; they are happy to have done an interview and then to never hear about the study again. Others, however, will appreciate finding how the study ended. At a minimum, I think it is good practice to send a thankyou letter.

Recording methods

Recording interview data in an organised and purposeful manner is fundamental to qualitative interviewing. It is one of the principal differences between interviewing for purposes of research and normal conversation (Lofland & Lofland 1984). There are a number of options available to researchers. Each of these is linked closely with the style of interviewing and the specific data requirement of your research questions (Lee 2004). For example, if the aim of an interview is to increase the researcher's familiarity with a particular setting or person, basic written memos may suffice. In contrast, interviews where the researcher wants to analyse the data, looking for themes, will require verbatim recording of all conversation and detailed records about body language and location (Facey 2003; Corbin & Strauss 1985).

Structured interviews usually have relatively simple data recording requirements as the interviewer simply ticks or marks pre-established response categories. The techniques described below apply largely to semi-structured, unstructured and informal interviews. Whatever methods of recording an interviewer uses, they *must* explain them to the interviewee and gain permission to use them before the interview starts.

Field notes

It is extremely difficult to write down exactly what people are saying while at the same time listening to them and responding appropriately. For this reason, I recommend that most interviews should be recorded, using a tape recorder (Lofland & Lofland 1995:86–7). However, field notes are a fundamental qualitative recording technique and their use is advisable, even if you are using an audio-recording technique (Sanjek 1990). In addition to noting what an interviewee says field notes can record the following:

1 Points of emphasis in an interview (i.e. issues that the interviewer or the interviewee felt strongly about).
2 Issues that you may want to refer to later in the interview.
3 Mood, tone and facial expressions, body language, clothing or uniforms.
4 Details about other people who may have come into the room or even sat down and joined in.
5 Impressions about an interviewee's home or workplace.

Field notes are also helpful for recording interesting things that the inter-viewee might say to you before or after the formal interview and for use after the interview when interpreting typed transcripts of tape record-ings. Some writers advise interviewers to refrain from taking notes during the interview in case it distracts the interviewee. It is often recommended that an interviewer sits down as soon as possible after the interview (e.g. when they return to their car) and write down impressions from the inter-view and things they want to remember (Berg 2004; Rice 1996). While I also recommend this practice, I have found that writing some notes during an interview is rarely disrupting for participants. It may even serve to encourage them by demonstrating your interest in their state-ments. Keep in mind, however, that writing notes during some moment of disclosure can stop the interviewee in their tracks.

Another technique I have recently adopted is to develop a simple document for recording background and demographic details. Lofland and Lofland term these 'face sheets' (1984:57). Face sheets record factual data about the interviewee relevant to the research project, such as age, name, sex, education, race or ethnicity, occupation and number of children. In studies with more than one interviewer, documents like this also provide a record of the name of the interviewer, the number of tapes used and other notes of that nature. I staple these sheets to any field notes taken during or after the interview. See Chapter Four for other advice regarding field notes.

Audio recording

The majority of semi-structured and unstructured interviews are tape-recorded, although digital recording appears to be replacing tape recording as the standard form of audio recording (see later in this section). However, tape recording is cheap, easy to use and familiar to most researchers (Warren et al. 2003:94). As long as you have access to a decent micro-phone (either integrated into the recorder or separate) the sound quality for tape-recorded interviews is usually fine (Grbich 1999:111). The most important thing is to audio-record interviews whenever possible:

> All kinds of data are lost without tape-recording [or other audio-recording]: the narrative itself, intonation, nuance, meaning and sequence. Some people will claim that in some instances tape recording is obtrusive, or is not feasible . . . these instances arise from time to time. But more often than not interviews lend themselves to recording without problems and most respondents when informed about the intended use and benefits of recording, agree to it. (Hermanowicz 2002:496)

When using a tape recorder, I like to use a separate microphone placed between the interviewer and the interviewee. This means that I can have the actual recorder close by and keep an eye on it fairly unobtrusively. The value of this will become apparent if tapes need to be turned over during the interview. It is advisable to use standard-sized cassettes instead of mini- or micro-cassettes. Standard cassettes have better recording quality than micro-cassettes. They are also stronger and more likely to survive the rewinding and fast-forwarding associated with transcription. Avoid voice-activated recording. The majority of tape recorders have this option, so ensure that it is turned off. It can make the tapes harder to transcribe because you have no idea about the length of pauses between speaking, and the recording may miss the first letters of some words. Most universities have requirements for the storage of research data, so tapes will need to be kept and stored under lock and key, *not* erased and used again.

Since the mid-1990s, various digital recording tools have become available to qualitative researchers. For example, MiniDisc recorders, recording directly onto a laptop computer, digital voice recorders and portable MP3 recorders (Maloney & Paolisso 2001). It is also possible to convert interviews recorded using a tape recorder to digital files that can be stored on a computer or a compact disc. This is usually achieved by linking a tape player with a computer or MiniDisc recorder via a cable and playing the interviews so they are re-recorded in a digital format. I have done this, and while it may be time consuming, the sound quality is fine.

These newer forms of digital recording have a number of advantages. They tend to have much greater sound clarity (Stockdale 2002). They are more flexible in terms of recording times, there is no need for bulky cassette tapes and digital files/CDs are easy to save for archiving. It is also possible to edit interview recordings using a computer, and digital recording may give you the option of easier transcription (Mitchell et al. 2004; Muhr 2000). Files can be emailed to other researchers or transcribing services. Once a research group, organisation or department has made an investment in digital recording, they are likely to find it cost-effective and convenient. However, there are a number of important issues to consider before adopting digital recording.

Newer tools tend to be expensive and may require access to additional equipment such as computers and software (Moloney & Paolisso 2001). If you are already involved in research or working in conjunction with experienced researchers, it will be important to ensure that any digital recording technologies are compatible with existing infrastructure, such as transcription devices, software (e.g. qualitative analysis software) and expensive external microphones. Newer versions of the major qualitative analysis software packages often accept digital files. These can then be transcribed within the software program. However, older ones may not, making it necessary to type the files up into a standard wordprocessing document.

Another issue to consider is the rapid rate of change in newer technologies. A case in point is MiniDisc recording. MiniDisc is gaining in popularity among qualitative researchers. The quality of recordings is greater than audiocassette, and discs can record for much longer amounts of time. MiniDisc players usually have an external microphone jack, and the recorders are small and lightweight. However, the format seems to be losing popularity among the companies that manufacture the technology in favour of 'solid state' technologies such as MP3 recorders. The cost of replacement or additional MiniDisc recorders is not coming down, and if they become obsolete, researchers will be left with discs that they cannot play.

A third issue to consider is portability and power. For example, recording onto a laptop provides excellent sound quality; however, laptops are heavy and bulky when compared to smaller tape recorders. In relation to power (as with tape recorders), ensure that any equipment you use is capable of operating on battery power.

Whichever type of audio recording is used, it is essential that the interviewer becomes familiar with their equipment prior to the interview. Practise setting up and using the equipment and become confident changing tapes, discs or memory cards, batteries and cables. I feel sick in my stomach when I remember mistakes I have made because I was nervous; for example, pressing Play instead of Record or plugging the microphone into the wrong socket. It is also a great deal less distracting for the interviewee if the interviewer isn't fussing over the equipment.

It is also important that you are aware of the range of your microphone. Microphones vary in this regard. Generally, I have found it useful to sit the microphone on a mouse pad or hand towel to cut down on vibration with the table. This is particularly relevant if you have to use an inbuilt microphone in a tape recorder as these tend to record the sound of the tape turning, if you lay them on a hard surface. Related to this point, rooms with carpets, curtains and soft furniture tend to produce better recording than large empty rooms with lots of hard surfaces.

Records and transcription

After deciding how to record interview data, decisions need to be made about precisely what information will be recorded. In terms of background data, it is usual to record the date and location for all interviews, and details of any participants. The usefulness of this type of information will become apparent if you ever conduct research that spans several years or conduct more than one research project at the same time.

When we move onto the actual interview, the 'gold standard' is full transcription. However, what this means varies from project to project. Generally, it means that the interview was either audio-recorded or a note-taker able to write very quickly recorded the entire interview. The audio-recording or full written notes are then transcribed to produce an interview transcript. This transcript will contain all conversation in the order it was held and possibly field notes as well. In methodological approaches that focus closely on the structure of verbal interaction (e.g. ethnomethodology), the transcript will also include all conversational pauses and filler sounds (Lynch 1993).

Transcription should occur as soon as possible after the interview. Grbich suggests that it should occur within 12 hours to maximise recall (1999:100). If your study is utilising methods such as member checking, ongoing iterative analysis or multiple interviews with each participant, make it a priority to keep on top of transcription as the material will be necessary to prepare for the next interview.

Transcription is an interesting process. In some projects – particularly inductive approaches, like grounded theory, or approaches where researchers are encouraged to immerse themselves in data, such as ethnography – the act of transcribing is viewed as a valuable and reflective stage. In these cases, it is inappropriate to have interviews transcribed by external agents, such as transcription services (as a note, on-line transcription services are available for data recorded using digital technologies).

Certainly I consider that transcription should be recognised as an analytical process (Ashmore & Reed 2000; Riessman 1993). When a person doing transcription is listening to a tape, they are making decisions about what an interviewee said and how they said it. Sometimes this interpretive process is straightforward and readily apparent; for example, when a word is barely legible or audible and the transcriber decides what the word was. However, it also occurs in less obvious instances, when the person doing the transcribing decides to emphasise a word or omit a pause. Translating verbal interaction into a document inevitably changes it subtly.

I didn't fully realise this until I gave some interviews to someone else to transcribe because I had run out of time. When I read over the transcripts, there were sections that seemed slightly different to how I remembered the interviews, and I had to listen to all of the tapes again (Hansen 2001).

Listening to the interview on tape while transcribing can be fascinating. I often notice things while doing this that I missed entirely during the interview (perhaps because I was busy thinking about my questions or worried about something else). For these reasons, I think it is better for the researcher to do their own transcription. If an alternative person does the transcription, then include them in other processes of analysis, if possible. The person doing the transcribing also needs to understand the importance of transcription to the research project. Stress that they should attempt to record exactly what they hear. Interestingly, having another person transcribe interviews can be useful if they then talk to you about the interviews and discuss their interpretations. It's a way of getting another viewpoint.

Transcription is painstaking work and takes a lot longer than you might expect. Roulston et al. (2003:656–7) also describe the difficulties associated with transcription. Their students described it as challenging, lonely and tiring. In our work, I usually expect one hour of interview tape to take up to four hours to transcribe. This varies according to the quality of the recording, the level and complexity of the details being recorded on the transcript, and typing speed.

Transcription machines are worth acquiring if your project has a large number of interviews. They are tape players with headphones, a foot pedal for fast forwarding or rewinding, and often a dial that allows you to slow down the speed of playback.

Many researchers use a process of selective transcription to save typing time. In practice, this means they listen to the tapes and then only type up those sections of the interview they think are important. This may mean omitting interview questions and any times when the interviewee was not directly addressing topics closely associated with the research questions. This process can have negative consequences:

1 A loss of conversational context – the role of the interviewee can be overly minimised.
2 Issues that may not seem important at the time may prove to be so later.

As such I do not recommend selective transcription for most projects. If it is necessary, then it is essential that the researcher does the transcription themselves so they are aware of how decisions were made about what to include and what to omit.

Interview guides and open-ended questions

As mentioned above, semi-structured interviews have lists of questions often called interview guides. While these are far more fluid and dynamic than questionnaires or structured interview question lists, they still require planning and careful consideration (Lofland & Lofland 1984:53). Researchers conducting unstructured interviews also need to plan some appropriate interview questions (Seidman 1998). However, unlike semi-structured interviews, these are not prepared before the interview. In reality, semi-structured interviews also require interviewers to construct questions 'on their feet'. This is often difficult for beginner interviewers, as normal conversation tends to include all of the types of questions best avoided in qualitative research interviews.

In qualitative interviewing, good questions are open-ended and never leading or overly directive. Open-ended questions encourage full responses, whereas closed questions often result in yes or no answers. The importance of asking non-leading questions is readily apparent. Questions such as 'Don't you think . . .?' or 'Don't you agree?' tend to put answers in interviewees' mouths and are unlikely to produce quality interview data. Roulston et al. (2003) found that novice interviewers have difficulty constructing open-ended questions and also tend to 'elaborate extensively, consequently forfeiting the clarity of the question' (2003:661).

In addition to being open-ended and non-directive, interview questions should reflect the issues of interest to the researcher as well as the types of language and issues of interest to the interviewee. This can be quite a difficult thing to achieve. Questions should not include theoretical or highly abstract concepts (such as 'surveillance' or 'social construction') and jargon unless the interviewee is also familiar with these. I have had trouble with this in the past as it often takes several interviews to realise that concepts or terms you have taken for granted are quite alien to the interviewees.

Also to avoid are two-in-one questions and 'why' questions (Grbich 1999:107). Two in one questions are difficult to answer, and the interviewee will often only address one part of the question. 'Why' questions tend to result in justifications from the interviewee. 'How' questions are more effective.

Many writers suggest that an interviewer begins with broad descriptive questions and follow with probing questions to elicit further detail (Lofland & Lofland 1984:54–6). Probes aim to encourage elaboration on a specific subject or to uncover or draw attention to what is not mentioned. Some probes are written on an interview guide to remind the interviewer to follow up certain aspects of the interviewee's narrative.

Notes might say, 'changes over time?' 'emotional tone? changes in importance?' (Lofland & Lofland 1984:57). Other types of conversational probing can be achieved via techniques. A powerful technique is sitting and waiting. Interviewees often pause to gather their thoughts. If the interviewer sits patiently rather than asking another question, the interviewee may continue and elaborate unasked. Other such techniques include taking the previous statement and turning it into a question, asking for examples and asking questions like: 'Was this what you expected?' 'How did you feel?' 'How so?' or 'How not?' Great interviews are characterised by the depth of detail from respondents.

> Meaning is typically the most problematic part of interviews, and is the monster that most eludes the beginning interviewer. People are inclined to be general rather than detailed – this is a common speaking convention. But like great conversations, great interviews reveal things previously unknown and often hidden . . . (Hermanowicz 2002:485)

Probably the most important rule of thumb when developing interview guides is to keep everything as short and simple as possible. A good semi-structured interview runs for between 60 and 90 minutes. Any longer than this is tiring, and an overly brief interview is unlikely to collect detailed data (Hermanowicz 2002:487). In my experience, an interview of this length can only support about 12 interview questions. It is difficult to provide an inclusive list of tips for interview guides, as the ideal interview guide varies from project to project. Listed below are strategies that I have found to be successful.

1   Attempt to weave questions into the interview in response to the interviewee instead of reading them out in the order they are written.
2   Ask questions that are interesting for the interviewee, that reflect their concerns.
3   Use soft, approving but relatively neutral sounds and gestures to indicate interest such as 'Mmm', 'Interesting', 'Can you tell me more about that?' or 'Yes'. These will encourage further discussion by the interviewee without distracting them or throwing them off track.
4   Probe by asking for clarification, details and examples; for example, 'How so?' 'Could you elaborate?' 'Tell me more about . . .'
5   Ask additional questions in response to interesting statements or issues made by the interviewee.
6   Note the things that are not being said; ask about these.
7   Remember that the interviewee can also ask you questions and that you should try to answer these. But keep it brief; after all, you want to listen to them.

Improving your interviewing skills

Because the interviewer is the most important data collection tool in interview-based studies, all researchers who conduct interviews need to become the most accomplished interviewer they can (Hermanowicz 2004). It is rather difficult to list the qualities of a skilled interviewer, as desirable attributes do vary according to the style of interviewing. The following list should be seen as a generalised guide rather than as all-encompassing.

Attributes of a skilled interviewer:

1 Able to develop trust and rapport.
2 Respectful and interested in the interviewee.
3 Allows the interviewee to schedule locations and dates for interviews.
4 Enjoys the interview.
5 Listens well.
6 Persistent.
7 Not afraid to be vulnerable themselves.
8 Responds to cues from the interviewee; for example, discomfort, frustration, tiredness.
9 Plans interviews suited to the needs of the interviewee.

Many health professionals have received training and are experienced in interviewing related to case-history taking or psychological counselling. However, such interview skills may need to be 'unlearnt' for qualitative research interviewing (Minichiello et al. 1990; Britten 1997). For example, those accustomed to interviewing for the purposes of taking case histories will need to ask less directed questions and give interviewees more time and control. Those accustomed to interviewing as part of psychological counselling may be highly skilled at building trust and rapport but unfamiliar with other types of interviewing that are not purposefully therapeutic (Whyte 1982). Morse and Field (1996:82) argue that health professionals who use counselling techniques during a research interview may inhibit the interviewee. For example, questions such as 'Are you saying that . . .?' or 'It seems to me that . . .?' make it easier for the interviewee to agree with the interviewer and close off the discussion rather than putting forward their own perspective (1996:82).

Because interviewing skills tend to develop with practice, the quality of interviews I conduct often improves over the course of a project. Certainly listening to recordings or reading transcripts from earlier interviews is a useful way to identify bad habits, such as interrupting people, discomfort with pauses or not listening well to the interviewee. Morse and Field (1996) also suggest that health professionals review transcripts from their interviews to improve their interviewing style. 'Problems are easy to spot in a typed transcript' (1996:82). The transcript from a successful interview will show that the participant did most of the speaking while the interviewer listened well, asked for clarification and encouraged the interviewee.

Roulston et al. (2003) recommend practising interviewing or conducting pilot interviews for the purpose of self-reflection and critique. This has a number of benefits. It facilitates the identification of the types of challenges that often occur during an interview-based study and gives an interviewer time to develop a response to these – for example, unexpected participant behaviours, disturbances during interviews, consequences of the interviewer's actions, emotional responses on behalf of the interviewer or interviewee, maintaining interview flow, phrasing and negotiating questions, and dealing with sensitive issues (Roulston et al. 2003:648–55).

Chapter summary

This chapter has provided an overview of qualitative research interviewing. It began with a short discussion about interviewing in general and recent shifts in the way that interviews are viewed by qualitative researchers. Four different styles of interviewing were introduced. These are structured interviews, semi-structured interviews, in-depth unstructured interviews and informal interviews. The practicalities of being an interviewer and planning interviews were outlined. The principles of qualitative interview questions and interview guides were described and advice was given on improving interview skills.

Interviewing is one of the most widely practised qualitative data collection methods (Seidman 1998; Atkinson & Silverman 1997; Britten 1997). It is a flexible and powerful data collection method. For example, it was used by Gahnstrom-Strandqvist and Josephsson (2004) to study interaction between occupational therapists and clients with a mental illness.

In studies where the researcher requires detailed information about the experiences, meanings and opinions of individuals, interviews are the most appropriate data collection method. However, interviews studies are labour-intensive and time consuming. They take a great deal of time to transcribe and are heavily dependent on the skills of the interviewer. As such, interviews are less suited to studies with large numbers of research participants. Too much interview data actually works against the type of detailed analysis that interview data requires. Some of the benefits of interviewing are clearly demonstrated in the following case study by Jon Adams.

Case study: In-depth interviews with GP therapists practising CAM

Dr Jon Adams, Director, Qualitative Research Laboratory, Faculty of Health, University of Newcastle, Australia

By the mid 1990s the mainstreaming of complementary and alternative medicine (CAM) (a range of therapies and diagnostics including acupuncture, aromatherapy, homeopathy and reflexology) in the United Kingdom was well under way. CAM was shown to be increasingly popular among patients, with the number of private CAM therapists rapidly growing and the medicines attracting significant interest from within the medical profession.

Early research established a small but not insignificant level of CAM practice among doctors (especially in general practice). Unfortunately, the vast majority of this work had been questionnaire based and there was a serious lack of in-depth and rich exploration of such integration from the experience of the doctors themselves. While social science had begun to explore the changing relationship between the medical profession and CAM, previous work focused upon the medical elite leaving the experiences of grassroots doctors unexamined.

In response, I set out to explore this area focusing research attention upon general practitioners (GPs) actively employing CAM within their National Health Service care. My main concern was to explore the under-standings and experiences of such GP therapists themselves. How were these GPs incorporating various CAM within their more conventional practice? How did the GP therapists make sense of and justify the practice of medicines not traditionally associated with medical training and in some cases contradicting biomedical science's understanding of the body, health and illness? How did the GP therapists appropriate their 'new' technologies and knowledge to the general practice setting? And how did their practice of CAM relate to their professional identity as a doctor more generally? In essence, this was a research adventure into the world of GP therapy, exploring the language of world members and, through careful questioning and listening, identifying the cultural cartography of this particular medical world.

It was decided to employ in-depth interviews with GP therapists practis-ing CAM. Twenty-five such interviews were eventually completed over a nine-month period. All interviews were conducted in the GPs' consulting rooms and lasted between one to two-and-a-half hours.

While the interviews were semi-structured (I employed a very rough theme list highlighting a number of general areas I wished to explore), I was very much cognisant of the need to allow the GPs the opportunity to fully express their own issues and concerns regarding their practice of CAM. As such, I invited self-directed exploration throughout the interview process and attempted to limit my input to simply help clarify and expand points and tease out particular issues.

A number of major themes emerged from these interviews. The doctors described the difficulties of practising CAM within their general practice. These included the problem of time – fitting therapies such as homeopathy, which can sometimes involve lengthy consultations into the busy and over prescribed general practice environment – and opposition from hostile and uncooperative medical colleagues and practice partners unwilling to support such 'fringe' medicines in general practice.

The GPs described how their integrated practice of CAM not only fitted comfortably within general practice but also expanded their vision and understanding of this particular field of medical care. The doctors appropri-ated their CAM use to the general practice setting through reference to the 'holistic' and 'patient-centred' nature of both styles of medicine (often contrasting their primary care to hospital medicine). In addition, a fear of what they saw as the 'movement' of evidence-based medicine (described as limiting their practice autonomy and disregarding their artistic and intuitive practice) further pronounced what they perceived as the need for CAM integration in primary healthcare. The doctors were also keen to distinguish themselves from CAM therapists practising outside the National Health Service and without medical training or qualifications. This 'style' of practice was demarcated as potentially dangerous and primarily based upon financial considerations rather than the best interests of the patient.

All these themes, among others, highlight the 'balancing act' facing these grassroots GP therapists. On the one hand, they are personally engaged in importing practices and technologies (not traditionally associated with their field of medicine) that they perceive as advancing and modernising the appeal of general practice. However, on the other hand, they run the risk of being too closely associated with these 'alternative' medicines and ultimately facing sanctions or excommunication from others in their professional world. The identification of such ongoing struggles for practitioner identity and territory not only contributes to the general understanding of CAM integration but also helps expand research attention beyond simply the approach and pronouncements of the medical elite regarding CAM. The qualitative inter-views provided an early exploration of the medical world of GP therapy from the perspective of those within, a world which has continued to expand and flourish to the present day.

Recommended reading

Fontana, A. & Frey, J.H. 1994, 'Interviewing: The art of science' in *Handbook of qualitative research*, eds N.K. Denzin & Y.S. Lincoln, Sage Publications, London pp. 361–76.

Gubrium, J. & Holstein, J. (eds) 2002, *Handbook of interview research: Context and method*, Sage Publications, Thousand Oaks, California.

Lofland, J. & Lofland, L.H. 1995, *Analysing social settings*, 3rd edn, Wadsworth, Belmont.

Mischler, E.G. 1986, *Research interviewing: Context and narrative*, Harvard University Press, Massachusetts.

Roulston, K., de Marrais, K. & Lewis, J.B. 2003, 'Learning to interview in the social sciences', *Qualitative Inquiry*, vol. 9, no. 4, pp. 643–68.

Seidman, I. 1998, *Interviewing as qualitative research: A guide for researchers in education and the social sciences*, Teachers College Press, New York.

six

FOCUS GROUPS

Focus groups collect data from group discussions around a focused topic. They are well suited to research projects requiring information about public understandings and social context (Kitzinger 1994). Focus groups usually consist of four to ten participants, a facilitator (also described as a moderator, or focus group leader) and a note-taker. The central feature of focus groups that differentiates them from interviewing (apart from the larger number of people involved) is the role played by interaction between the participants (Rice & Ezzy 1999:73). Researchers who use focus groups hope that the group processes associated with focus groups will assist the participants to clarify and explore their views (Kitzinger 2000).

Focus groups have been used to investigate a wide range of health-related issues (Barbour & Kitzinger 1999). Examples include the experiences of mothers caring for children with cancer (Clarke et al. 2002), the experiences and learning during a graduate nurse program (McKenna & Green 2004), and barriers to the provision of care for people with dementia (Hansen et al. 2005). Focus groups are particularly popular in research investigating experiences, attitudes and opinions. For example, Seymour et al. (2004) conducted focus groups with 32 older people to explore their views on advance care statements and planning for the end of life. They recruited focus group members from 11 different community groups. The authors chose focus groups as their primary data collection method because they considered that group discussions with similar people would help participants to explore the sensitive issue of end-of-life care (Seymour et al. 2004:60). They found that focus group discussion did help to open up discussion. Similarly, Gilliam et al. (2004) held seven focus groups with young Latina women attending a contraceptive outpatient clinic to identify their perceptions and attitudes about contraceptive side-effects. Focus groups were found to be valuable in this study because they facilitated the type of anecdotal discussion about contraception that was favoured by the young women.

Background to focus groups

Like interviews, focus groups are a data collection method that can be adapted to suit a wide range of different types of qualitative research projects. Researchers working within different methodological traditions have adapted focus groups to suit their needs (Morgan 1997). As a result, focus groups range from formalised quasi-scientific events aimed at producing 'objective' results for market research to the extremely flexible consciousness-raising group meetings associated with some feminist action research (Morgan 1997; Stewart & Shamdasoni 1990).

Focus groups were originally developed as a data collection tool for social research during World War II. They were used by Robert Merton to investigate how audiences were receiving military training films. Audience members were asked why they had responded positively or negatively to certain aspects of the film. Unlike the other methods being used to measure this at the time, focus groups allowed for open-ended questions and exploration of the reasons why audience members responded favourably or negatively (Merton 1956). However, despite Merton's successful work with focus groups, the method was not adopted by other social scientists for several decades. Focus groups were next used in the fields of market research and political polling to trial products and to investigate consumer opinions of advertising, people and products (Barbour & Kitzinger 1999). They became the predominant data collection method in this field and have remained popular (Nucifora 2000).

Despite the popularity of focus groups in marketing research, they were not adopted by academic qualitative researchers until the 1980s (Berg 2004:125; Hamel 2001). The use of focus groups in health-related research developed alongside the growing popularity of qualitative research in the 1980s and '90s; in particular, action research and feminist traditions. Focus groups have been used successfully in health-related studies investigating attitudes and knowledge towards illness and medical care and for health education (Rubin 2004; Sussman et al. 1991; Basch 1987). More recently, researchers have started using focus groups to investigate illness and professional narratives and stories (Flaherty et al. 2004; Jordens & Little 2004). Focus groups are also used as an initial stage in the process of developing new questionnaires

(O'Brien 1993). In these instances, focus groups are used to trial possible questions and terminology with a group of people similar to the intended recipients of the questionnaire.

Focus groups are popular in qualitative health research for several reasons. They are valuable in situations where the researcher has only a limited amount of time to gather data from one group of participants or setting (Berg 2004:123). Focus groups are also seen by many researchers as creating a safe environment for the sharing of experiences and for facilitating 'participation' in research (Baker & Hinton 1999; Montell 1999; Morgan 1997). Because of this, some researchers describe focus groups as a useful method for exploring sensitive issues and for accessing groups who may be 'otherwise relatively marginalised in research' (Seymour et al. 2004:60). It needs to be recognised, however, that it is much harder to ensure confidentiality with focus groups than it is for interviews. Another potential drawback is that an overly dominant, judgmental or aggressive participant could easily deter other participants from speaking about sensitive issues.

The group interaction associated with focus groups also provides a number of advantages. It allows researchers to observe and listen to how participants speak with each other and how they respond to each other's views. This may include jokes, teasing, arguing and colloquial language. Group interaction may also lead to participants challenging each other or raising new issues previously unthought of by the researcher and some of the participants. In focus groups, the goal is to let people spark off one another, suggesting dimensions and nuances of the original problem that any one individual might not have thought of (Rubin & Rubin 1995:140). This is a useful way to stimulate discussion and may also have a 'quality-control effect' where participants check each other's statements. Listening and speaking with each other may assist participants to clarify their points of view (Bates et al. 2004; Denning & Vershelden 1993). For this reason many participants come away from a focus group feeling that they have learnt new things from other group members. Furthermore the experience of telling others about aspects of their lives and experiences can be pleasurable and empowering for participants (Morgan 1997).

Despite the many advantages of focus groups, they should not be viewed as an easy alternative to interviews. They collect a quite different type of qualitative data and do not allow for in-depth exploration. Furthermore, focus groups tend to be costly, complex to organise and time consuming to analyse.

Selecting and recruiting focus group members

To a large degree, the sampling required to address a research question or questions will operate as the guide when choosing focus group participants and deciding how many focus groups to run. Focus groups seem to run well with between five and eight participants. Larger focus groups can become unwieldy and smaller focus groups may not provide enough momentum to stimulate discussion (McLafferty 2004). While there are no set guidelines on the best number of focus groups to include in a study, this decision should be made on the basis of collecting enough data to achieve the aim of the focus groups and pragmatic reasons such as the amount of time and funding available. Focus group data is complex and may take longer to transcribe and analyse than interview data. Morse recommends that final decisions about the number of interviews or focus groups in a study should be made part-way through the project, allowing the researcher(s) to assess the amount and quality of data already collected (Morse 1991, 2000a).

Focus group composition

Focus group members are often linked by a shared characteristic. Examples are gender, ethnicity and a shared experience, background or occupation. This linking characteristic will often be closely related to the focused topic or issue. Focus groups can be held with strangers or with 'naturally occurring' groups, such as colleagues or members of a support group (Kitzinger 2000). When focus groups are held with heterogenous groups, the members may have very different experiences or opinions that will trigger debate and interest. However, these types of groups may require greater moderator intervention (McLafferty 2004).

In projects where focus groups are being conducted in order to familiarise the researcher with a new setting or group of people, it is most useful to select focus group members who know a great deal about the situation and who are 'articulate, wise, knowledgeable and helpful'. These participants will act as key informants, or guides (Lofland & Lofland 1984:43).

The style of discussion is very much affected by the focus group participants and their relationship to each other. Morgan (1997) argues that careful sampling is vital for an interesting and lively discussion. Participants who haven't ever met each other before will have an extremely different focus group in comparison with a focus group where the participants have longstanding relationships (e.g. from working in the same ward of a hospital or community nurses in a small rural community). It is also important to recognise any hierarchies within the group. This is quite likely to occur in healthcare settings; for example, between physicians and nurses from the same hospital or physicians and their patients (Kitzinger 2000).

Recruitment

Recruiting for focus groups can be quite difficult. Accessing the people you want to speak with and then arranging for them to be available at the same time is never easy. If you have ever recruited for interviews and discovered how difficult it can be to line up one person for an interview, just imagine trying to get as many as eight people in one place at the same time. The type of study and the people you are trying to recruit will affect how you recruit. It will generally be easier to arrange for focus groups with pre-existing groups. The following strategies have proven useful when recruiting for focus groups in my own research:

1 Approach people directly.
2 Send a letter of invitation followed by a phone call.
3 Ask their peers or friends to contact them first.
4 Use professional groups, phone books and so on to locate people.
5 Advertise in newspapers, on notice boards, in newsletters etc.
6 Conduct focus groups with people already participating in your study.
7 Offering incentives for participation, such as coffee vouchers, food or a gift (not money).

As with recruiting for other data collection techniques, some rules of thumb apply. Always follow up a letter of invitation with a phone call within a relatively short amount of time. Interest wanes quickly, and many people interpret a slow reply as a sign that the researcher is not interested or does not value their time. Thank all possible participants who contact you, even if they don't participate.

Location and set-up

Focus groups have quite stringent requirements in terms of location. If the location is unsuitable, it will impact negatively on the quality of data you are able to collect. It may also hinder your attempts to recruit. There are a number of things to look for in a good focus group location.

Transport and access are two key issues associated with successful recruitment. The focus group must be easy for participants to travel to and to get in and out of. It may be necessary to consider wheelchair and pram access, parking and access to public transport. The researcher who is organising the focus groups may need to drive participants to the focus group location and then home again afterwards. In addition to physical access, the timing of focus groups will impact on whether participants actually attend the group. Some participants may have minimal free time or only be available in the evenings.

The location needs to be safe for the researchers and the participants. Most researchers will be covered under some type of insurance associated with their workplace or academic institution; however, you still need to think carefully about safety. For example, if you are running a focus group on a university campus of an evening, will participants feel safe to walk back to their parked cars? If you are running a focus group for people who may engage in a potentially illegal or stigmatised activity such as intravenous drug use or domestic violence or who suffer from an illness that inspires strong emotion in others, will they feel comfortable about attending the location you have chosen, particularly if the focus group is known to be discussing that topic?

As with any group activity that may run for some time, focus group participants, the facilitator and note-taker will need access to toilets plus somewhere to prepare drinks and a light meal or snack. While on the subject of food, I have found it far better to eat before a focus group than to offer participants food when the focus group is under way. Having food available during the focus group tends to break people's concentration and stops them from talking. Good options for pre-focus group snacking include coffee/tea and muffins, fresh fruit, nuts, water and fruit juice.

Most importantly, a focus group needs to be held somewhere where you will not be disturbed. Nothing disturbs concentration and makes participants feel self-conscious more than people knocking on the door or walking through the room. I have also found that a small stuffy room sends everyone to sleep very quickly. The room needs to be sufficiently large and to have either air conditioning or windows that can be opened.

Suitable venues should also be amenable to audio recording. This may range from a purpose-built room with inbuilt microphones and video recording facilities to a quiet room with access to power points and space on the table to set up a microphone. If you are conducting your research in association with a university or government department, it is worth asking around to see if there is a room with inbuilt recording facilities. Because focus groups are likely to be audio-recorded, it is also beneficial if the room has soft surfaces rather than hard ones; hard surfaces tend to create harsh sounds on the recording.

In terms of seating, focus groups require a large table surrounded by chairs. I think the table and chairs are important. This set-up keeps people focused and paying attention. It also seems to make participants feel comfortable – the table serves as a type of shield but also facilitates intimacy as people lean towards each other when speaking. I once conducted a focus group in a typical loungeroom with armchairs and a sofa. While it was certainly comfortable, I found it was too easy for participants to 'zone out'. It also felt rather strained as people were sitting at different heights and quite a long way back from each other.

There are many places where you will be able to find a suitable location for a focus group. Any type of building set up for the public, such as government offices, local council chambers, doctor's surgeries, schools, universities and libraries will usually have a room set aside for meetings. These can often be booked or hired for a small fee.

Facilitation/moderation

A moderator, or facilitator, supports the group and ensures a successful conversation takes place. Their role is to keep the group focused, listen closely and to occasionally ask questions that stimulate discussion. While facilitators are often described as focus group leaders, in most instances they actually need to minimise their participation in the focus group discussion in order to maximise interaction between the focus group participants. At times, however, they may need to control the group or an individual. It is important for a moderator to explain their role to participants at the beginning of the focus group.

The moderator/facilitator role

Much has been written about the facilitator/moderator role (MacDougall & Baum 1997; Stewart & Shamdasoni 1990). Their role is not to judge participants' responses or to express their own opinion. Instead, they need to listen closely, be open-minded, observe the interaction and attempt to create opportunities for all participants to express their views. At times it can be useful for the moderator to adopt various strategies to stimulate discussion. For example, playing devil's advocate, offering an alternative point of view, asking an individual a direct question and using conversational probes (MacDougall & Baum 1997; Denning & Verschelden 1993). It is important that the moderator has sufficient understanding of the research project. This allows them to judge whether or not the focus group is producing the types of information required and helps them to formulate appropriate questions in context. A moderator should be sensitive to the needs of participants, non-judgmental about responses, respectful, open-minded, knowledgable, a good listener, demonstrate leadership and observational skills while also being patient and flexible (Rice & Ezzy 1999:85)

It is often difficult to find a balance between overly directive leadership and letting the group slip away from the desired topics into a discussion about something completely different. It is also challenging trying to encourage quieter members of the group or dealing with a particularly dominant participant. Another challenge that often arises occurs when members of a focus group address their talk to the moderator rather than interacting with each other. This may be necessary in the early stages of a focus group as the members may not feel comfortable speaking with each other until they have had time to gauge each other's views. However, it is not desirable for an entire focus group to consist of participants answering questions put by the moderator. Kitzinger (2000) recommends that facilitators try to take a non-interventionist stance in the early stages of a focus group and then ask more direct questions to urge debate and to encourage participants to discuss 'inconsistencies between participants and within their own thinking' (2000:4).

Moderation/facilitation styles

Every focus group is different. Consequently, moderation styles may need to be changed from group to group. Stewart and Shamdasoni (1990) argue that the composition of the group and the purpose of the research will necessitate particular styles of facilitation:

> For example a less structured and free wheeling approach to focus groups would be desirable if the purpose was to generate new ideas or to encourage creativity. On the other hand, a more structured approach with occasional in-depth probing may be required when the objective . . . is to generate research hypotheses or to diagnose potential problems with a new program, product or service, particularly when the topic is sensitive or potentially embarrassing. (Stewart & Shamdasani 1990:74)

As with qualitative interviewing, moderation is a skill that improves with practice. I have observed also that it is a skill that lapses when not used. For this reason, you may find that your moderation skills improve over the duration of a project. It is usually preferable for a researcher to collect their own data. However, there are times when another person is better suited to facilitate your focus groups. Times when it may be appropriate to train another or additional person to moderate focus groups for your project are listed below.

1 Instances when the researcher does not speak the language well or at all. In this case, other researchers have found training a native speaker to facilitate often works better than using a translator (Rice & Ezzy 1999:77).
2 Studies with a large number of focus groups.
3 When it seems appropriate to have a moderator who participants can easily relate to or feel comfortable with (e.g. if you are male researcher and want to run focus groups for breastfeeding mothers, it might be useful to have a female moderator).
4 When the researcher is closely involved with the focus group participants.

Questions and prompts

The questions presented to the focus group by the facilitator are important because they focus the discussion on topics and issues related to the research questions and they set the tone for interaction. As with qualitative interviews, open-ended questions are preferable as these encourage broad responses and 'allow respondents a great deal of freedom to provide the amount of information they want to give' (Stewart & Shamdasani 1990:74). Stewart and Shamdasani distinguish between primary and secondary questions. Primary questions introduce new topics or areas of discussion. Secondary questions follow up primary questions and may act as probes encouraging clarification and expansion from the participants (1990:75).

Grbich (1999:112) describes three strategies aimed at producing focus group discussions. She recommends trying one and seeing how the group responds. If that strategy does not seem to be working, then an alternative can be introduced. The first strategy is termed the 'circle technique'. It requires the facilitator to ask each participant the same question in turn. While this may not produce much variation in the data, she describes it as a useful way of breaking patterns of dominance if one or two focus group members are taking over the conversation. It may also be a useful strategy at the beginning of a focus group to get participants talking. The next strategy involves throwing out 'one exciting or controversial idea' and observing the outcome (1999:112). The third strategy is a type of brainstorming where the facilitator presents a scenario of ideas and the group develops a response.

Faciliators may also have considerable success using visual strategies or by taking along unusual objects for participants to touch and discuss. These could include pictures, advertisements, a series of statements on large cards, or a medical instrument such as a speculum (Chui & Knight 1999; Easthope 1997; Kitzinger 1990). Kitzinger (2000) describes a successful and dynamic focus group on breast cancer where a participant removed her prosthetic breast and handed it around the group. She also describes another useful visual technique. This involves the use of statements, pictures or words written on large cards. A colleague of mine used this technique when she ran focus groups with retired high school teachers. She described it as being highly successful (Easthope 1997). The cards may be used in a number of different ways. The facilitator can hold them up and ask the group to comment. Alternatively, the group can be asked to sort statement cards into groups along an agree/disagree continuum. Kitzinger (2000) has used this method with various focus groups; for instance, midwives exploring their views of their professional responsibilities, people discussing understandings about HIV transmission, and older people talking about residential care. The discussion arising from this method is likely to be of more interest than the final arrangement of cards. This strategy is a good 'ice-breaker' that encourages interaction between the participants. Blank cards can also be taken into the group and then, towards the end of the group discussion, filled in with key phrases or words arising from the main points raised by the group. These cards can be shown to the group for their comments.

Recording focus group data

As with other qualitative data collection methods, it is vital to record focus group data in a systematic and comprehensive manner. Qualitative researchers should never make the mistake of relying entirely on their memories or assuming that brief notes will suffice (Berg 2004; Morse & Field 1996). It is highly unlikely that any researcher will be able to easily distil and identify the important and relevant aspects of the 'social events unfolding or the words being spoken before them' without time and reflection (Lofland & Lofland 1984:46). Following on from this, the aim of a good researcher is to record as much of the data as carefully as possible. Three methods are commonly used to record focus group data. These are note taking, audio recording and video recording.

Note taking

When a note-taker is used in a focus group, they sit in an unobtrusive location and record details as specified by the researcher. They need to be introduced to the participants at the beginning of the focus group but after that they should fade into the background. The type of notes they take is determined by the study design and the needs of the researcher(s). For example, because I usually tape-record focus groups, I have found it to be useful for the note-taker to record the name of each speaker and the first word they utter. In this way, an abbreviated transcript is produced that allows for much easier full transcription of an audio recording.

A note-taker can also act a little like an observer. They might record details of the room and its lay-out, major topics raised, the mood or feel of the group, emotions or actions, and their own responses to the focus group as it progresses. It is important to discuss with the note-taker the type of notes you want taken before the focus group. If you are conducting a project with more than one focus group, obtain feedback from the note-taker about the note taking after each focus group. They may have suggestions or need to tell you that the type of notes you asked for were too difficult to produce.

Audio recording

Most focus groups are recorded, using a tape recorder or a digital recording device, such as a MiniDisc player or an MP3 recorder. As with interviews, there are a number of different options for recording voices in a focus group. With focus groups, the key issue to remember is that you are recording a large number of people and they will probably be sitting around a table. Therefore, you will need a top-quality microphone with a wide recording radius, such as a flat-bed microphone, or lapel microphones. Another option is to use a purpose-built room with ceiling microphones.

Video recording

Video recording of focus groups has a number of advantages. When used in conjunction with audio recording, the video record is extremely helpful in identifying which participant said what when transcribing the audio recording. Video also captures non-verbal communication and allows for a permanent record of group interaction and behaviours. As such, it may remove the need for a note-taker. Grbich (1999:113) recommends that the video recorder be placed at some distance from the group. It is important to recognise, however, that videotaping a focus group may lead to difficulties in ensuring confidentiality.

Ethics and focus groups

Apart from the usual ethical concerns of any research project, the biggest ethical issues that seem to arise with focus groups are problems of confidentiality and anonymity. When numerous people are involved, it is difficult to ensure that participants do not gossip about the participants in the group. Focus groups need to follow the usual ethical procedures for your workplace or academic institution. In addition to these, participants should agree to respect each other's confidentiality. An option used by some researchers is to ask participants to sign a document stating that they understand the importance of confidentiality and agree to protect the privacy of all the focus group participants.

Problems can also arise if one participant behaves badly towards another. The focus group moderator has to feel comfortable in reining in an out-of-control participant; for example, if one participant bullies or tries to dominate another or starts to say aggressive or antagonistic things.

Chapter summary

Focus groups are a highly flexible and adaptable qualitative data collection method. They allow researchers to explore an issue or topic in a relatively short amount of time through group interaction. This acknowledges the socially embedded and contextual nature of understandings, experiences and attitudes (Kitzinger 1994:117). Focus groups have been used successfully in a wide range of qualitative projects exploring topics ranging from sensitive issues – such as contraception, sexuality and drug use – to people's views about health professionals and workplace changes.

This chapter began with a background section describing the history of focus groups and why they are popular in health-related research. Next the pragmatic aspects of organising and running focus group were described. This included recruitment, choosing group members, selecting a location and recording data. The next section of the chapter focused on focus group facilitation and focus group questions. The final section addressed the major ethical issues associated with focus groups.

Focus groups are often difficult to arrange (Rice & Ezzy 1999:91). However, in my experience they are usually well worth the effort. For example, in my doctoral research I conducted interviews with medical doctors (Hansen 2001, 2003). The interviews went well, and I decided not to run any focus groups. More recently, I ran two studies in which medical practitioners were involved in interviews and focus groups (Hansen et al. 2003, 2004). I then became aware that listening to doctors speaking with each other is noticeably different from listening to them speaking to a non-medical interviewer. They often challenged each other or asked for clarification. In addition, I learnt a great deal about the terminology they were using and about the ways that medical doctors interact with each other. I saw how they were reluctant to appear ignorant in front of their peers and so at times gave quite different descriptions of their practice to those they had given to me in interview. Conversely, being around their peers also seemed to break down some of the conventions about doctors presenting a confident front to non-medical people. For instance, when one doctor in a particular focus group admitted that they didn't know much about the disease we were discussing, this produced similar disclosures from other focus group members.

The value of focus groups as a qualitative data collection method is also demonstrated below in a case study from Kevin Dew, who conducts qualitative research in the area of public health.

Case study: Focus groups about perceptions of earthquake risk

Dr Kevin Dew, Senior Lecturer, Social Science and Health, Department of Public Health, University of Otago, New Zealand

Although you may think that public health research, with its foundation in epidemiology, is a hard-line quantitative discipline, in fact qualitative research is playing an increasingly important role in this area. This is particularly the case for certain areas of public health research, such as the social determinants of health, health-services research and health promotion. My current research projects involve me working alongside health professionals, such as GPs and psychiatrists. In one project we are exploring the complex issues related to healthcare delivery in mental health, and in another we are looking at interactions between patients and professionals in order to shed light on the decision-making processes related to the rationing of healthcare resources.

I am also in the fortunate position of supervising a wide range of postgraduate theses in public health and related areas (e.g. bioethics and primary care) where the collection of qualitative data lies at the heart of the research. Many of the students I supervise are health professionals. As such, much of the research I am involved in, and the theses I supervise, entail an element of multidisciplinary research. Much of the fun of this research is the intellectual engagement across disciplines and worldviews, and the challenges that are posed in these engagements. In all cases the health professionals have concluded that the use of qualitative research, and the engagement with a sociological perspective that I bring, has been enriching. In turn, my increased understanding of the world of the health professional and the issues they face have enhanced my analyses. The potential for misunderstandings and the difficulties of overcoming our pre-determined notions about what constitutes appropriate research should not be glossed over, but we have always gained a more comprehensive view of the research process in the end.

The research discussed here was undertaken by two social scientists, although with input at important times from public health researchers and earthquake scientists. Our research topic was the perception of earthquake risk and responses to that risk. Very topical, given that the research was conducted in the earthquake-prone city of Wellington. The research included a survey of earthquake scientists about the way their research was represented in the media and a telephone survey of the public where we explored a wide range of issues. These included respondents' perceptions of earthquake risk, what could be done to prepare for earthquakes, what they had done to prepare for earthquakes, and what sources of information they trusted. Then we used focus groups to explore issues raised in the previous components of the research.

We had a number of issues we wanted to explore in the research. I was particularly intrigued to find that there was a high level of distrust of earthquake scientists. Why should this be so given that earthquake scientists had no obvious commercial or political ties? We also wanted to explore people's thoughts on why many respondents who had quite a good knowledge of what they could do to prepare for an earthquake had not acted on that knowledge.

The participants for the focus groups were selected from survey respondents who said they would be available for the focus groups. The organisation of the focus groups was not an easy matter. Finding enough people who were willing and able to come on the times we had available took some co-ordination. We supplied coffee, tea and biscuits, and two of us were involved in conducting the focus groups. I facilitated the focus groups and my colleague, Tony Mangan, made sure the recording equipment was working and took notes. Before the focus groups started there were nervous moments waiting to see if anyone would turn up. Invariably, fewer turned up than we expected, but we had good size groups and got some excellent material. There was also the tricky time when some participants had turned up and we were waiting for others. During this time we made sure the consent forms were signed and tried to engage in light social pleasantries while avoiding any discussion of the research topic until we turned on the recorder.

To kick the discussion off I decided that we should use an icebreaker that would hopefully engage everyone in the conversation. Quite by chance there had been a few minor earthquakes in the week or two before the focus groups were held, and so I decided to ask people what they did when they felt the earthquake. The earthquakes occurred in the early hours of the morning so everyone was in bed at the time. This icebreaker worked brilliantly. Not only did most people have something to say, but also the topic lent itself to humorous responses that had the effect of relaxing everyone. Some people slept through it, some woke to hear their husband's snoring, some sat up in bed waiting to see if it was going to be the 'big one'. But not only did the icebreaker work as an opening gambit for the rest of the 'real' discussion, it became of interest in itself. In all but one or two cases, participants did nothing when the earthquake awakened them. So this led to the question of why they did nothing. And what would make them do something? Overall, the focus groups were a lot of fun and worked tremendously well. When listening to the tapes it was very tempting to analyse the data not for the content (what people were saying) but for the interaction and interplay between the participants – an obvious possibility being a gender analysis.

However, it was not all plain sailing. When we invited participants to attend, we offered them transport to the focus groups if they did not have a car. Only one person took this up, and she lived quite far away. I dutifully picked her up and brought her along – adding more difficulty to the pre-focus group arrangements. It was a little annoying when the person I picked up refused to participate in the discussion. Questions directly addressed to her were usually met with a shrug of the shoulders. Then about half an hour into the focus group she stood up, moved to the side of the room and lit up a cigarette (which was actually breaking the local laws on smoke-free workplaces). I did not know what to do. I did not want to disrupt the focus group too much, and I did not want to seem authoritarian and order her out of the building. I looked pleadingly at the participants for some sign about how to respond – and thankfully they just nodded their heads to signal that it was OK, let's just get on with it.

In retrospect, it may be that this person volunteered because we had said that all participants would go into a draw with a prize of $50. One of the highlights for the research was taking a $50 cheque to one of the prize-winners – an elderly lady who lived in very humble accommodation, and who was so excited at winning (she had never won anything in her life, she said) that tears came to her eyes.

A number of important issues came out of the focus groups, including the suggestion that preparation campaigns needed to take into account that New Zealanders were no longer the DIY lovers of old, and so very simple instructions on how to do things to the house to prevent earthquake damage were important. The focus group material was included in a report that went to the Earthquake Commission and in a paper published in the *New Zealand Journal of Media Studies* (Dew 2001). Among other things the latter article explored the issue of trust in science, and suggested that a lack of trust is not simply an outcome of a lack of knowledge by the public, but can be seen as a pragmatic response to uncertainty of science and the sensationalism of the mass media. Since the completion of that project I have been involved in a number of other research projects where focus groups have been used. After that initiation I can say that I am less worried about how many turn up – and I look forward to analysing focus groups because the data is so rich. Even if you get only two showing up, which happened to me on one occasion, you can still get important insights (though you might have to call it a dyad interview instead of a focus group). All in all, the focus groups were a very satisfying experience from a research point of view, and were great fun to boot.

Dew, K. 2001, 'On shaky ground: Earthquake experts and the media', *New Zealand Journal of Media Studies*, vol. 8, no. 1, pp. 3–18.

Recommended reading

Barbour, R. & Kitzinger, J. (eds) 1999, *Developing focus group research: Politics, theory and practice*, Sage Publications, London.

Kitzinger, J. 1994, 'The methodology of focus groups: The importance of interaction between research participants', *Sociology of health and illness*, vol. 16, issue 1, pp. 103–21.

Krueger, R. 1994, *Focus groups: A practical guide for applied research*, 2nd edn, Sage Publications, London.

Morgan, D. 1997, *Focus groups as qualitative research*, 2nd edn, Sage Publications, Newbury Park, California.

Qualitative Health Research 1995, Special Issue: Issues and application of focus groups, vol. 5, issue 4.

seven

ANALYSING QUALITATIVE DATA

Analysis is the process by which qualitative data, such as interview transcripts, field notes and documents, is transformed into results, such as new understandings, theories and statements about the empirical world. Raw data alone is little more than piles of transcripts or field notes. For qualitative data to become meaningful, a researcher needs to sift through it and identify issues of importance to the research project. How a researcher chooses to 'make sense' of the data they have collected is closely linked with the research questions, their disciplinary background, the theoretical approach underpinning the research project and personal choices related to preferred modes of work.

There are numerous different approaches to analysing qualitative data, and considerable variability exists between researchers in how they apply these approaches. Furthermore, very few of these approaches have clearly established 'methods'. Instead, they are better understood as focusing devices or as different ways of thinking about qualitative data and identifying interesting and important patterns in data as related to a particular research project. The lack of clearly developed methods of data analysis and the large choice of approaches available can make analysis an extremely confusing process for novice qualitative researchers searching for answers about the 'best' or the 'right' way to 'do analysis'.

Four approaches to analysing qualitative data are discussed in this chapter. These are content analysis, iterative/thematic analysis, narrative analysis and discourse analysis.

The chapter closes with a case study from Douglas Ezzy. He describes the emotional aspect of analysing interview data, drawing on examples from a project investigating the relationship between religiosity and living with HIV/AIDS.

Background

Qualitative data analysis reflects the close relationship between data and theory in qualitative research. There are no hard and fast 'rules' for how qualitative data should be analysed. Instead, there are a number of loosely defined approaches that have been developed by researchers working within the various theoretical perspectives underpinning qualitative research. These approaches act as data filters and reflect underpinning assumptions about what is important in qualitative data and how this can best be obtained through research. Some of these approaches have been used and described so many times that they have become a recognised approach. For example, grounded theory is an example of the iterative/thematic approach to data analysis. There is consistency among researchers who conduct grounded theory (Strauss & Corbin 1990). However, there is also considerable variation among qualitative researchers who describe their preferred approach to analysis as being iterative/thematic (or discourse analysis or narrative analysis etc).

As with data collection, debate and pluralism characterise qualitative data analysis. 'What links all the approaches is a central concern with transforming and interpreting qualitative data – in a rigorous and scholarly way – in order to capture the complexities of the social world we seek to understand' (Coffey & Atkinson 1996:3). While it is possible to collect qualitative data with little or no reference to theory, it is extremely unlikely that a researcher unfamiliar with theory will develop a well-designed research plan. As the research problem, research questions and methodology guide data analysis, it will be difficult to conduct meaningful and rigorous analysis that is likely to be accepted for publication or to receive a high grade in university assessment without some reference to theory. Furthermore, placing your work within the larger frameworks provided by theory allows a researcher to make a more effective contribution to wider bodies of knowledge through their research:

> The practice of some researchers of refusing to consult the literature and refusing to place the theory within the context of work that has already been published, is a serious problem. It results in a plethora of small and competing contributions to the literature. These contributions are not additive, they do not build on what has been published before; thus, qualitative inquiry as a discipline makes only a minor impact and has trouble demonstrating its contribution to science. (Morse 2000b:715)

The first two approaches discussed in this chapter are content analysis and iterative thematic analysis. These fall within a 'realist' perspective to qualitative data, where researchers aim to elicit 'some external reality', such as experiences, facts or events (Silverman 2003:343). This is a perspective familiar to most health researchers as it reflects ideas about research that underpin scientific medical knowledge. Content analysis began as a basic statistical research method used to count the number of times certain words and phrases were used in press coverage and wartime propaganda (Krippendorf 1980). After World War II, researchers from a range of disciplines, including linguistics, psychology, sociology and history, used content analysis when analysing texts. This led to a broadening of scope for content analysis where the context of certain words or phrases was seen as important, and images were also included as units of analysis (Mostyn 1985). Researchers tend to be attracted to content analysis because it is seen to utilise a number of features more commonly associated with quantitative research, such as criteria of reliability and the capacity for research to be replicated (Mayring 2000; Grbich 1999:224).

Iterative thematic analysis entails identifying 'themes' in data. Themes can be thought of as recurring patterns of interest in the data (Burnard 1991). Areas of interest are suggested by the research problem, the research questions and a desire to formulate hypotheses or propositions. Iterative thematic analysis has a long tradition of use in sociology, anthropology, philosophy, nursing, public health and applied health research. It is also the approach to qualitative data analysis used in many qualitative evaluations (Adams et al. 2003; Patton 1990). Iterative/thematic analysis is clearly located at the heart of the interpretive sociological tradition (Adib Hagbaghery et al. 2004; Brett et al. 2002; Martin et al. 1999).

Researchers conducting an iterative/thematic analysis consciously move between analysing and collecting new data in 'the field' and analysing and reflecting on data they have collected. This approach is particularly conducive to a flexible research design where patterns and themes identified in data already collected are used to re-focus or adapt research questions and data collection tools, such as interview guides or focus group questions. Researchers conducting an iterative/thematic analysis use a variety of techniques to identify 'interesting' sections in the data. Coding is the best known of these techniques. Coding involves identifying sections of the data, marking them (coding) and then sorting these sections in groups of like and unlike etc. Precisely how researchers code their data is strongly influenced by their training and the particular type of thematic analysis they are using. A well-known type of thematic analysis is grounded theory (Strauss & Corbin 1990; Glaser & Strauss 1968). Grounded theory is an approach designed to allow researchers to generate or discover a theory. It uses systematic coding procedures known as open coding, axial coding and selective coding (Strauss & Corbin 1990). Open coding is the first stage of coding. It involves breaking the data into identifiable properties, categories and dimensions. The researcher searches for 'differences and similarities between events, actions and interactions' and applies labels to them (Rice & Ezzy 1999:195). The next stage in the analysis is axial coding. This type of coding is about making connections between categories (Dey 1999:2). During selective coding, the analyst attempts to integrate and order their analysis, using core headings. For example, Jack et al. (2005) used a grounded theory approach to develop a theory of maternal engagement with public health nurses and family visitors in Canada. They collected data through a review of client records and 29 interviews with clients. The major themes identified in their study related to maternal engagement with home visitors were overcoming fear, building trust and seeking mutuality. Within each of these, the authors identified a number of sub-themes. For example, under the category of overcoming fear, the authors identified a number of strategies used by mothers such as 'hiding nothing', 'trying to measure up' and 'protecting self' (2004:185).

In contrast to content analysis and thematic analysis, narrative analysis and discourse analysis are both methods associated with postmodern, poststructuralist and feminist theoretical traditions. They represent a 'linguistic' or 'textual' turn in qualitative research that became apparent in the 1970s and onwards. Both approaches focus on the ways that research participants – and this includes the researchers – use language to 'generate plausible accounts of the world' (Silverman 2003:343).

> The ways language produces and constrains meaning, where meaning does not, or does not only reside within individuals' heads, and where social conditions give rise to the forms of talk available. (Burman & Parker 1993b:3)

In contrast to realist approaches like thematic analysis and content analysis, where researchers are trying to get to the 'truth' of the matter or trying to identify processes, experiences or 'reasons' why people behave or respond in a certain way, researchers using narrative or discourse analysis are interested in how stories and discourses are used by research participants to produce an account that is convincing and satisfying to them and to the researcher (Williams 1984). They may also be interested in what this story or account might indicate about the social and political realm. Accordingly, researchers working with narrative and discourse analysis are as interested in how something was said and perhaps the reasons why it might have been said in this way as they are in what was said. In narrative research in particular, researchers are also interested in the ways that people's ideas about how and why something happened shape the reality of their illness or experience of medical procedure (Frank 1995).

> According to narrative theory, by producing narratives about themselves, patients, in collaboration with their doctors, may make sense of their condition . . . narratives may be used to configure present and future experiences, in addition, by telling stories patients can provide doctors with information that places their medical condition in the context of their everyday life. (Martin et al. 1999:80)

Narrative analysis as an approach is a newcomer when compared with content analysis and thematic analysis. While narratives in myth and texts have long been the focus of literary theory, an explicit interest in narrative has only been apparent in qualitative analysis conducted as social research since the 1970s. The development of a narrative approach reflects an increasing interest among qualitative researchers in the ways that people's ideas and language are situated in social and historical contexts. Traditional realist approaches are seen by some researchers as failing to 'account for the insistence with which certain stories or explanations are put forth, take hold and shape images' (Sacks 1996:59). Rice and Ezzy argue that 'narrative analysis is distinguished from other forms of qualitative data analysis by its attention to the structure of the narrative as a whole' (1999:125). Some particularly interesting qualitative studies in health have made use of a narrative approach. For example, Patricia Bailey's study of breathlessness in patients with chronic obstructive pulmonary disease (Bailey 2004), Deborah Lupton's study of doctors (1997) and Waitzkin's et al. (1994) study of ageing and medical encounters.

Discourse analysis is a critical approach where researchers focus on qualitative data such as interview transcripts, newspaper articles or textbooks as 'texts' (Lupton 1992). Texts are seen as reflections of wider processes of power and discourses. Burman and Parker (1993b:4–7) describe three reference points or areas of focus that characterise different approaches to discourse analysis. These are an interest in conversational repertoires, the 'making of sense', and the relationship between discourses and social relationships. A type of discourse analysis derived from the work of Michel Foucault and poststructuralism (Fox 1993; Foucault 1980) is perhaps the most widely applied type of discourse analysis in health research. This type of discourse analysis has been particularly popular in nursing, social work and public health. Examples of health-related projects using this type of discourse analysis are Nick Fox's study of power relations between surgeons and anaesthetists (Fox 1992) and Sarah Nettleton's study of dentistry in the twentieth century (Nettleton 1992).

Deciding how to analyse data

In qualitative research, the collection of data and analysis of data often occur concurrently. As data is collected, researchers start analysing and interpreting it (this process actually begins 'in the field' during data collection). It addition, lulls in data collection serve as valuable opportunities for a researcher to focus on its analysis. Analysis often continues long after data collection is completed.

> This sequential analysis or interim analysis has the advantage of allowing the researcher to go back and refine questions, develop hypotheses, and pursue emerging avenues of inquiry in further depth. Crucially, it also enables the researcher to look for deviant or negative cases; that is, examples of talk or events that run counter to the emerging propositions or hypotheses and can be used to refine them. (Pope et al. 2000:114)

Analysis is an integral aspect of the overall research design and something that you should be considering during the early stages of developing a methodology and a project plan. However, as with other aspects of qualitative research, you may change your mind about the analysis in response to the data or shifts in the project's focus. This was discussed in Chapter Two. When deciding on how to analyse your data, you need to consider the following.

The theoretical background of your project

The wider discipline in which you are working (e.g. nursing, sociology, education, psychology) and the particular theoretical and hence the methodological framework of your project will impact on the analysis options available. The goals and objectives of analysis are closely related to the methodology for the project.

> Some (for example phenomenology, grounded theory, discourse analysis) seek to create new understanding and theory from data. In some (such as

some field studies and ethnography, action research and pattern analysis), the goal is rich description and vivid presentation of new understanding. (QSR 2002:10)

Type of data to be collected (methods and volume)

Some types of analysis are better suited to certain types of data. There are also historical traditions associated with certain data collection methods and analytic approaches. Furthermore, data needs to be maintained in certain forms for different types of analysis. For example, thematic analysis of interviews requires full interview transcripts and cannot be done using hand-written field notes alone. Content analysis of large amounts of data is greatly aided if you can scan documents into a computer. This means that before you even collect data, you need to know the format required for the type of analysis you plan to use.

Purpose of the research

If you are evaluating a health program for a funding body as compared to exploring indigenous discourses of Western biomedicine for a Masters project, you will find that your options in terms of types of analysis are quite different. Evaluation as a discipline tends to be conservative and, consequently, utilises a fairly small group of qualitative analytic techniques. By contrast, academic research is generally speaking more adventurous, provided you embed your choice of analytic approach within the relevant literature. You will have many options available to you. Other factors associated with the purpose of your research that will influence your choice of analytic approaches include:

1 The audience for the results, including publication.
2 Time available.
3 Resources available, including skilled people, access to software and computers.

It is possible to use more than one approach to analysis on the same data in the same project. However, the results from different types of analysis are not always comparable. For example, content analysis and iterative/thematic sit easily together. They are both realist. Attempting to conduct an iterative/thematic analysis and a discourse analysis on the same data in the same project would be complex in terms of the language and ideas available to the researcher, their capacity to draw conclusions and problems associated with writing up the results.

Beginner and less experienced researchers have a tendency to combine qualitative analysis approaches without adequately acknowledging the epistemological origins and assumptions that underpin the methodologies they are blending. This is poor scholarship and it is also confusing for the readers of their research (Cheek 2000; Morse & Field 1996). I am not arguing that a researcher should never use more than one approach in the same project. Rather, if researchers do this, they need to acknowledge any problems related to combining approaches and be clear in their own minds about what they are doing and why they chose to do it in that particular way. Their justification and discussion of these issues needs to be clearly articulated and included in the write-up.

Some disciplines and individual researchers are strongly opposed to combining different analytic approaches in the same project. However, different approaches to qualitative data analysis can also be viewed as different ways of helping a researcher gain insight into the phenomena under study. This is something that you will have to judge for yourself after reading in your field and consulting with your colleagues and research supervisors.

To complicate matters further, the lines between different types of analysis are often ambiguous. Many researchers construct personalised approaches to qualitative analysis that merge various aspects of the approaches outlined in this chapter. Working with the various approaches inevitably changes how a researcher thinks about research and data. For example, I have tended to use iterative/thematic analysis for much of my health-related research. This reflects my training in fairly traditional sociology and the fact that I find this type of analysis is well accepted by my medical colleagues. However, the way I conduct an iterative/thematic analysis has been moderated by other approaches to analysis because my research practices have been strongly influenced by feminist and postmodern writings. Accordingly, my personal approach to iterative/thematic analysis relies heavily on several key features of discourse and narrative analysis; for example, an interest in language, social and historical contexts and power structures, as well as a focus on researcher reflexivity. In addition, over the last year I have been learning how to use a purpose-built software program designed to assist with analysing qualitative data. Working with this program is further changing the ways that I approach and manipulate data and altering my approach to conducting an iterative/thematic analysis.

Using computers

Whatever analytic approach you use, there are two main aspects of qualitative data analysis. One is actually interpreting the data in some way, and the other is keeping track of it and physically manipulating it (Knafl & Webster 1988:196). Until relatively recently, the mechanics of data manipulation were done by hand, using pens, paper, scissors, glue and string (marking transcripts for coding, filing, sorting sections of data, typing field notes, searching for examples and counting occurrences). However, as personal computers became readily available, word processing and database software packages were used to assist with these tasks. There are also purpose-built software packages designed for qualitative data analysis. These include NVivo, NUDIST, Atlas ti and The Ethnograph.

Computers have revolutionised the ways that qualitative researchers manage their data, making it possible for them to manipulate data in increasingly sophisticated ways and often in smaller amounts of time (Fielding & Lee 1998). This in turn can assist with better interpretation and associated conceptual activities:

> Benefits of computer programs [include] saving time for the researcher, saving space for file management, and reducing the manual labour required by the more traditional methods of cutting, pasting, sorting and storing. These savings free the researcher to invest more time and energy in the analytic process. (Taft 1993:381)

Skilled users of certain software packages find that the way they interpret data actually changes because of the increased options offered by the software (Gibbs 2002). 'Software for qualitative data analysis can benefit the researcher in terms of speed, consistency, rigour and access to analytic methods not available by hand' (Weitzman 1999:1241). However, computers and software packages are tools; the actual interpretation and decision making about the relative importance and meaning of patterns in the data is something that only the researcher(s) can do. It is also very difficult to use computers effectively without some training in qualitative analysis and an understanding of qualitative methodology.

Some concern about computer-aided analysis is apparent in the qualitative research literature (Kelle 1995). Commonly discussed issues include worry that the programs may encourage a methods-obsessed approach to qualitative data analysis, where researchers design projects to suit programs rather than seeing programs as a tool to assist analysis (Tesch 1990:324). Another issue is the fear that using computers for analysis may impose a false sense of 'objectivity' and reification of conceptual artefacts like codes and themes because researchers are able to conduct complex searches that sound similar to statistical analysis and to produce complicated looking diagrams, tables and even graphs. By performing all of their analysis on a computer, researchers also risk distancing themselves from their data and data from its social context (Fielding & Lee 1998; Aljunid 1996; Taft 1993; Seidel 1991).

The various purpose-built qualitative analysis software packages are designed to assist researchers with particular approaches to analysis and therefore particular methodologies (i.e. ethnography, phenomenology or grounded theory). The two types of analysis that are best suited to the packages currently dominating the market are content analysis and thematic analysis. However, researchers wanting to conduct narrative analysis and discourse analysis can make use of some software packages to assist with managing large amounts of data and to aid close textual work. Newer versions of software packages have been designed with greater flexibility, in order to be more useful to researchers who want to use a range of analytical approaches.

Computer-aided analysis using purpose-built software is not necessary for small projects with only a limited amount of data. Here the advantages of using a computer are limited. However, if your project is large, or if there are multiple researchers (or students) or research sites, I recommend using a program to help sort and organise your data. Even when using a software program, I find it helpful to conduct initial reading and reflection on data using printed transcripts and handwritten field notes – these evoke memories of data collection and remind me that producing data even to this stage has involved researchers and participants in an interactive and therefore interpretive process.

Because there are so many packages available – as well as new programs coming onto the market and existing programs being revised regularly – making a decision about which package will best suit you is difficult. I suggest that decisions related to choosing a particular program focus on the purpose and aims of the research and pragmatic issues associated with how much time you have to learn a new program, financial costs and availability. Unfortunately for Macintosh users, the availability of programs is sorely limited.

It is best to choose a flexible and relatively simple-to-use program. These tend to be newer programs or newer versions of existing programs. It is desirable to choose a program that has readily available training and on-line or telephone support for users. I have also found it helpful to choose a program currently being used by colleagues so that they can act as a users' support group. In a related issue, find out if your university or institution is currently supporting a particular package. They may be able to arrange access for you via a site licensing arrangement. It is also helpful to consider the following questions posed by Weitzman (1999:1251):

1   What kind of computer user am I?
2   Am I choosing for one project or for the next few years?
3   What kind of project(s) and database(s) will I be working on?
4   What kind of analyses am I planning to do?
5   How important is it to you to maintain a sense of 'closeness' to your data?
6   What are your financial constraints when buying software and the hardware it needs to run on?

Interpretive content analysis (counting occurrences)

Content analysis involves selecting units of analysis (i.e. what you are going to look for) and counting the frequency of these units in the data. These could be particular words or utterances in interview data or behaviours or types of clothing in an observational study. Content analysis is generally used when documents are the primary type of data; however, it can also be used for other types of data, such as observation data, interview data or media, such as film or magazines. Content analysis can be used in conjunction with another type of analysis. This provides numerical data in a study that might otherwise seem overly descriptive to readers more familiar with quantitative research.

Content analysis can be seen as a quasi-statistical form of qualitative analysis or it can be conducted in an openly interpretive way. The first type of content analysis requires that the units of analysis be fixed and concrete. Consequently, the units being counted are seen as having an objective quality – for example, counting the number of times a particular word or term is used in a text, or counting how many photographic images of women occur in a magazine.

> In general qualitative analysis does not seek to quantify data. Qualitative sampling strategies do not aim to identify a statistically representative set of respondents so expressing results in relative frequencies may be misleading. Simple counts are sometimes used and may provide a useful summary of some aspects of the analysis. (Pope et al. 2000:114)

In an openly interpretive content analysis, the role of the researcher as an interpreter is more explicit because they decide what constitute examples of a particular unit of analysis, possibly following an earlier thematic analysis. The units of analysis are often looser and more open to interpretation. In addition, the location of certain terms or phrases is considered to be important. The researcher decides what will count as an occurrence and then codes the documents accordingly. For example, in a study investigating how male and female bodies are represented in magazines, a possible code would be 'physically powerful female bodies'. The researcher would search the magazines for examples that they consider fit this code then mark them accordingly. The number of times this code was marked would be tallied.

As you can imagine, content analysis can be used to test a hypothesis; for example, that magazines aimed at women of different ages will reflect different leisure activities and levels of sporting involvement. Or that men and women are associated with different sports and leisure activities.

Researchers often use a qualitative analysis software package for content analysis as these packages allow the researcher to mark not just the word/phrase etc but also to record its context. The use of computers drastically shortens the length of time needed to conduct a content analysis.

Examples

Downe-Wamboldt, B. 1992, 'Content analysis: Method, applications and issues', *Healthcare for Women International*, vol. 13, pp. 313–21.

Evans, L. & Davies, K. 2000, 'No sissy boys here: A content analysis of the representation of masculinity in elementary school reading textbooks', *Sex Roles*, vol. 42, nos. 3–4, pp. 255–70.

Fields, E. 1988, 'Qualitative content analysis of television news: Systematic techniques', *Qualitative Sociology*, vol. 11, no. 93, pp. 183–93.

Gahnstrom-Strandqvist, K., Josephsson, S. & Tham, K. 2004, 'Stories of clients with mental illness: The structure of occupational therapists' interactions', *Occupation, Participation and Health*, vol. 24, no. 4, pp. 134–43.

Iterative/thematic analysis (identifying themes in the data)

Unlike content analysis where the researcher decides what they are looking for and then searches for this in the data, iterative/thematic analysis is largely inductive. While the researcher will inevitably have some ideas about what might be going on from their own experiences, their reading and training, thematic analysis stems from a tradition of qualitative research where the researcher attempts to be guided by the data rather than a pre-established hypothesis. In keeping with this, the researcher generally approaches the data as it is collected with a fairly open mind (although they are guided by the research questions) and attempts to identify important themes emerging in the data. In grounded theory, particular emphasis is placed on the importance of being guided by the data rather than being guided by ideas from the literature or existing theory (Dey 1999).

> Initially the data are read and reread to identify and index themes and categories; these may centre on particular phrases, incidents or types of behaviour. Sometimes interesting or unfamiliar terms used by the group studied can form the basis of analytical categories. (Pope et al. 2000:114)

Iterative/thematic analysis has two important characteristics. The first is the iterative aspect and associated 'data immersion'. The term iterative means repeating. The iterative aspect of thematic analysis is the way that the researcher repeatedly moves between different aspects of their research – collecting data in the field, transcribing and reading the data, reflecting and interpreting and then collecting new data (Grbich 1999:231). This process often lasts a considerable period of time and is very 'hands on'. Associated with the iterative process is an idea stemming from ethnography, that the researcher should immerse themselves in their data. In an effort to become closely acquainted with the data, many researchers consider it important to collect and transcribe their own data as well as reading and reflecting on it. This increases familiarity and expands a researcher's ability to make connections between different aspects of the data.

Associated with iterative/thematic analysis is a technique where researchers alter the focus of the research or the way they are conducting their fieldwork in response to the ongoing analysis of data already collected. Researchers may alter their interview guides, decide they need to interview a different group of people or start collecting new types of data. This highly fluid iterative process often continues until the researcher considers they have reached a point of data saturation where no new discoveries are occurring.

The second important characteristic of iterative/thematic analysis is the use of coding. Coding is a term given to marking interesting sections or 'chunks' in the qualitative data so that they can be identified and sorted.

Exactly how researchers use coding varies enormously. Highly systematised approaches, such as grounded theory, have clearly defined methods of coding, as mentioned briefly above (*see* Strauss & Corbin 1990 or Dey 1999 for detailed descriptions of these). Other researchers develop their own approach from project to project. Examples of the type of 'interesting' chunks that researchers often identify and mark in their data include actions, objects, key phrases or words, emotions, events, processes.

Coding helps a researcher to notice new things in their data by changing their relationship to the data, facilitating a process of reflection and discovery. Codes are a tool used by researchers; they are changeable and help a researcher to notice interesting things in their data and to gather sets of these together. The researcher can perform coding by writing on hard copies of transcripts or by using index cards. It can also be done using a computer. Interview and focus group transcripts are imported into the computer and then read on the screen and marked with codes. Coded sections of data can then be retrieved and sorted. The process of iteration and coding data and identifying themes is summarised below (adapted from Grbich 1999:234).

1 Collecting data and ongoing analysis.
2 Reading and reflecting on the data and developing and adding codes, as a way of indexing and sorting the data.
3 Refining codes through reading/reflection comparison/sorting. This stage of the process can be highly systematic or more loosely structured depending on your preference. This stage of analysis can be greatly assisted by using computer software that allows for quick searches and retrieval of data.
4 Developing some type of classification scheme or typology (this may be completely new and based solely on the data or it may be informed by theory or other research; it may be very ordered or relatively unstructured).
5 Searching for examples that don't fit the scheme; critically evaluating, adjusting, altering the scheme in response to these (this can be a long, ongoing process).
6 Re-examining typology in an attempt to generate propositions. Re-examining these in new ways, looking for complexity, associations etc.
7 Deciding on the key findings and writing these up; relating them explicitly to the research questions and the literature; illustrating this with many examples from the data.

An issue that is often debated among researchers who use an iterative/thematic approach to analysing qualitative data is how to avoid reaffirming one's own assumptions/biases. A number of solutions to this problem has been developed. Some writers suggest that researchers overcome overly subjective or potentially biased interpretations by making use of more than one analyst (Freeman & Sweeney 2001; Daly, McDonald & Willis 1992). Daly et al. (1992), in their study investigating the diagnosis of cardiac normality, made use of external researchers and also had cardiologists review the analysis and some of the empirical data: 'Our aim was to inter-pret the use of the test directly from the accounts of the actors themselves and not from any preconceived rationale of the use of the test' (1992:192). Using more than one analyst and devising ways to check the analysis of one researcher against that of others is a useful technique for some researchers and some research projects. However, the openly interpretive nature of iterative/thematic analysis means that 'the appropriateness of the concept of inter rater reliability in qualitative research is contested' (Pope et al. 2000:115; Armstrong et al. 1997).

Another way qualitative researchers avoid producing an overly narrow or 'biased' analysis is by reading widely. This means the researcher reads in the field, and across fields, comparing their interpre-tations with the results of other studies, both substantive and theoretical. They include reference to this process in the write-up of their work (Coffey & Atkinson 1996:140).

A third and complementary solution is to include in your write-up plenty of clear examples from the data which demonstrate the context of the themes etc that the researcher has identified. This allows readers to gauge the quality and reliability of the analysis for themselves. Personally, I have also found that when actually conducting the analysis, it helps to work with full transcripts on a regular basis rather than working only with already coded data that may have become separated from its larger context. This forces me to be aware of the informant's overall point of view and the important roles played by the interviewer and the analyst.

Examples

Corbin, J. & Strauss A. 1985, 'Managing chronic illness at home: Three lines of work', *Qualitative Sociology*, vol. 8, no. 3, pp. 224–47.

Davies, S. & Nolan, M. 2004, '"Making the move": Relatives' experi-ences of the transition to a care home', *Health and Social Care in the Community*, vol. 12, no. 6, pp. 517–26.

MacFayden, L., Amos, A., Hastings, G. & Parkes, E. 2003. '"They look like my kind of people" – perceptions of smoking images in youth magazines', *Social Science and Medicine*, vol. 56, pp. 491–9.

North, D., Davis, P. & Powell, A. 1995, 'Patient responses to benzodiazepine medication: A typology of adaptive repertoires developed by long-term users', *Sociology of Health and Illness*, vol. 17, no. 5, pp. 632–50.

Orona, C. 1990, 'Temporality and identity loss due to Alzheimers Disease', *Social Science and Medicine* vol. 30, pp. 1247–56.

Narrative analysis

A narrative analysis focuses on the ways informants use stories or narratives when talking or writing about their lives and opinions. Some studies explicitly set out to use narrative as a way of investigating and exploring the understandings of others. These studies are often interview-based, and the interviewer may use techniques designed to facilitate storytelling (Rosenthal 2003). In other studies, a decision to focus on narrative is made only after the researcher has started collecting data. As they reflect on the data, the importance of narrative in participants' accounts becomes apparent (*see* Williams 1984; Ezzy 1998; Rice & Ezzy 1999:120–1).

Content analysis and thematic analysis both break qualitative data down into smaller sections. Researchers using a narrative approach focus on the ways that research participants tell stories and avoid fragmenting their data through coding. Coffey and Atkinson describe the difference between thematic analysis using coding and working with narratives as follows: 'In turning from coding to narrative, we began to explore not only what was said in our data but also how it was said . . . a narrative approach can help to alert the analyst to research problems . . . that coding and content analysis may not uncover. A concern with narrative can illuminate how informants use language to convey particular meanings and experiences' (Coffey & Atkinson 1996:83).

David Silverman (2003) describes this attention to how respondents describe their worlds as an alternative to the realist types of analysis more commonly favoured by qualitative researchers (such as thematic analysis), where the researcher aims to accurately access the experiences and lives of their respondents in an attempt to 'index some external reality' (2003:343). In contrast to this endeavour, a narrative approach aims to 'open up for analysis the culturally rich methods through which interviewers and interviewees, in concert, generate plausible accounts of the world' (Silverman 2003:343). Narrative accounts can be analysed linguistically or sociologically. A linguistic focus pays particular attention to the use of language and structures within the narratives. A sociological approach focuses more on what the types of narrative told can tell us about the ways that the research participants have experienced their lives and the narratives available to them (Richardson 1990:24).

Borone (2001) argues that stories can act as a stimulus for discussion, as analysing stories can challenge common assumptions. Narrative-focused studies may also have positive characteristics for research participants. For example, Rosenthal (2003) conducted narrative-focused research with survivors of concentration camps and refugees. She considers that the act of describing their lives was beneficial for research participants. Another wonderful example of a narrative analysis is provided by Gareth Williams' influential 1984 paper on narrative reconstruction in chronic illness.

Williams (1984) conducted interviews with a number of people with rheumatoid arthritis. He was interested in their beliefs about the causes of their illness. As he interviewed people and reflected on the interviews, Williams decided that an individual's beliefs about their illness only made sense within the context of the larger stories they told about their lives. The meaning of their illness to them and the reasons why they believed the illness had occurred were inextricably linked with their narratives about 'their changing relationship to the world in which they live and the genesis of illness within it' (Williams 1984:175). Therefore, a narrative approach was the only way to fully understand their aetiological stories. An approach like iterative/thematic analysis, aiming to identify common themes across a number of interviews, would give a limited picture that may have been misleading.

Narrative analysis is an exciting way to take advantage of the richness of qualitative data and it allows the researcher to gain (and to convey to readers of their write-up) insight into the beliefs, action and values of participants, from within their own frame of reference (Grbich 1999:16). As qualitative researchers in search of insight into our social world, stories are fundamental to our work. It is important that we take time in interviews to ask informants about their stories. Understanding our data in terms of stories is a recognition that the issues/instances that emerge in our research are not isolated but in fact are embedded in peoples' lives, and that their understandings of their lives are constructed through language and interaction.

> Narratives focus on the details of the story and emphasise the context dependant nature of the particular story told. Narratives change depending on who tells them and ambiguity is a central part of a good story. (Rice & Ezzy 1999:119)

If you are interested in narrative analysis, there are a number of options available to you. You could begin your study with a focus on narrative. This would involve deliberately conducting semi-structured or unstructured interviews, using techniques of narrative interviewing (Bailey 2001; Clandinin & Mconnelly 1999). An example is asking questions aiming to elicit narrative, such as, 'Please tell me/us your family story and your personal life story/ I am interested in your whole life/ we have as much time as you like to tell it/ I won't ask you any questions for now' (Rosenthal 2003:917). Alternatively, studies might evolve into narrative-focused projects even if they did not start this way. If the existing data is marked with examples where participants have used storytelling to provide information about a topic or experience, these can be recognised in the analysis by focusing on narratives rather than themes and avoiding breaking interviews up into smaller and smaller pieces. Narrative aspects to the data can be further 'brought out' in the results through the use of life stories or case studies. These will demonstrate that the particular event being discussed cannot be understood outside its context within that person's life. Finally, a researcher can set out to formally study narratives, using one of the existing frameworks stemming from literary/historical theory (Bruner 1990, 1991; Bailey 2001) – for example, studies of plot structure, identifying elements of story structure.

Examples

Bailey, P.H. 2001, 'Death stories: Acute exacerbations of chronic obstructive pulmonary disease', *Qualitative Health Research*, vol. 11, pp. 322–38.

Clandinin, D.J. and Connelly F.M. 1999, *Narrative inquiry: Experience and story in qualitative research*, Jossey-Bass, San Francisco.

Clark, J.A. and Mischler, E.G. 1992, 'Attending to patients' stories: Reframing the clinical task', *Sociology of Health and Illness*, vol. 14, no. 3, pp. 344–71.

Frank, A. 1995, *The wounded storyteller*, University of Chicago Press.

Mischler, E. 1984, *The discourse of medicine: Dialectics of medical interviews*, Cambridge University Press, Cambridge.

Mischler, E. 1986, *Research interviewing: Context and narrative*, Harvard University Press, Cambridge, Massachusetts.

Williams, G. 1984. 'The genesis of chronic illness: Narrative reconstruction', *Sociology of Health and Illness*, vol. 6, no. 2, pp. 175–200.

Discourse analysis

The term discourse analysis is used to refer to a variety of approaches that focus on data as spoken and written texts (Gee 2005). Discourses can be defined as 'dynamic dialogues in which meaning is socially and histori- cally produced, reproduced and transformed in interaction' (Grbich 1999:153). 'Text' refers to a 'representation of any aspect of reality' (Cheek 2000:64). Discourse analysis can be described as 'a broad theor- etical framework concerning the nature of discourse and its role in social life, along with suggestions about how discourses can best be studied' (Potter & Wetherell 1987:175). Researchers using discourse analysis as an approach to guide their analysis of qualitative data are not focusing on the meanings individuals ascribe to their actions or their lives. Nor are they attempting to illuminate subjective experience or provide detailed descriptions of the empirical world. Instead, they are interested in the ways that problems and issues (e.g. health, disease, gender) are textually mediated through sets of largely taken-for-granted assumptions called discourses and the ways that 'language produces and constrains meaning' (Burman & Parker 1993b:3).

> The 'text' is merely a repository and a reflection of other processes. The experiences of those who produced them, or who are named therein, are not of particular interest except for their clarification of these wider processes of power and their help in exposing discursive practice. (Grbich 1999:152)

Discourse analysis draws on a range of disciplines, including psychology, philosophy, literary theory, sociology and linguistics. The discourse analysis conducted by researchers working in each of these fields varies in terms of emphasis and methods. As with other types of analysis, indi- vidual researchers often develop their own style of discourse analysis drawing on a range of features from different disciplines. Some researchers focus most heavily on the mechanics of how language is used (Nunan 1993). Others focus on the ways that language is used, enabled or constrained in some way and what this tells us about the sociopolitical situation and the relationship between discourses and wider processes of power 'that are socially and historically produced, reproduced and trans- formed in interaction' (Grbich 1999:153). These studies have explored the ways in which textual representations of gender, disease, illness, patients, healthcare practitioners etc are 'indicative of wider knowledge, belief and value systems' (Lupton 1994b:73). For example, powerful people or groups are able to make use of discourses or promote certain discourses that serve their interests (Gill 1993). For example, Ong and Glantz describe how discourses of 'junk science', 'sound science' and 'good epidemiology' are used by tobacco companies to discredit evidence that secondhand smoke causes disease (Ong & Glantz 2001:1749). Much of this type of discourse analysis is strongly influenced by the theorist Michel Foucault (Lupton 1992; Cheek & Rudge 1994). Foucault argued that knowledge is closely linked with power and so cannot be considered as objective or value-free. He also wrote about the important role of medicine as a force that shapes 'the beliefs and conduct of the population' (Nettleton 1991:99). Accordingly, discourse analyses drawing on Foucault tend to focus on 'issues of power, ideology, dominance, hegemony, inequality, and the production and legitimation of forms of knowledge that have enabled certain individuals, groups or ideas to dominate social processes' (Grbich 1999:151–2).

Because the ways that people understand the world, experience and behave is shaped by language, other researchers have focused on drawing out connections between discourses and behaviours (Plumridge et al. 2002). For example, a study of smoking cessation by elderly people with smoking-related illness found that participants able to access discourses where smoking cessation was described as achievable were far more successful than those who did not (Parry et al. 2001).

> . . . discursive constructions (having 'no choice' and getting 'another chance') used by the respondents position them in a way that constrains behaviour by closing down the option of smoking and/or opening up the possibility of change. In each telling, the respondents' (non-smoking) identities are confirmed anew, and this affirmation may assist in sustaining the change and provide protection against relapse. (Parry et al. 2001:481)

If you are interested in using discourse analysis as an approach to guide the analysis of qualitative data, there are a number of factors to keep in mind. The first is that such an approach sits particularly well with research projects informed by poststructural or postmodern theories. The second is that there is no 'method' or 'recipe' for conducting a discourse analysis (Cheek 2000:51). Cheek describes poststructural and postmodern approaches as 'ways of thinking about the world that shape the type of research that is done and the types of analyses that are utlized' (2000:4). The best way to learn how to 'do discourse' analysis is to read reports from other projects that use this approach. However, several authors have described the key features of a discourses analysis (Gee 2005; Cheek 2000; Parker 1992). Cheek (2000:52) describes the following practices:

1 Closely reading the text looking for evidence of discourses.
2 Paying particular attention to different levels of meaning and alternative perspectives.
3 Marking interesting sections and considering these in relation to the writing and research of others.
4 Investigating how discourses have been shaped, and which values and ideologies appear to be underpinning them, and tracing these historically.
5 Looking for evidence of challenges to discourses.

Examples of discourse analysis

Ainsworth-Vaughn, N. 1995, 'Claiming power in the medical encounter: The whirlpool discourse', *Qualitative Health Research*, vol. 5, no. 3, pp. 270–91.

Cheek, J. 2004, 'At the margins? Discourse analysis and qualitative research', *Qualitative Health Research*, vol. 14, no. 8, pp. 1140–50.

Cheek J. & T. Rudge 1994, 'Webs of documentation: The discourse of case notes', *Australian Journal of Communication*, vol. 21, no. 2, pp. 41–52.

McKie, L. 1995, 'The art of surveillance or reasonable prevention? The ease of cervical screening', *Sociology of Health and Illness*, vol. 17, no. 4, pp. 441–57.

Chapter summary

Analysis requires time, reflection and skill. 'Qualitative research requires the researcher to ponder and reflect on the data collected so as to find the meaning within' (Hunter et al. 2002:388). Researchers develop increasingly sophisticated techniques and styles of analysis over time. This reflects wider reading, practice, exposure to alternative approaches, life experience and increased knowledge about the research problems and qualitative research in general. Less experienced researchers often learn a great deal from working with more experienced researchers and seeing how they analyse qualitative data (Shelby 2000). Computer software packages are a useful tool to assist those researchers working with larger amounts of data; however, they are less useful in small studies and they cannot 'do the analysis' for a researcher.

This chapter provided an overview of four approaches to qualitative data analysis often used in health-related research. These are content analysis, iterative/thematic analysis, narrative analysis and discourse analysis. Each approach was explained, and examples of studies using the approaches were provided. The following case study from Dr Douglas Ezzy provides a discussion about analysing interview data in a qualitative study investigating the experiences and meanings of people living with HIV/AIDS.

Case study: Analysing interview data

Dr Douglas Ezzy, Senior Lecturer, School of Sociology and Social Work, University of Tasmania, Australia

In 1997 I was working at the National Centre in HIV Social Research, studying the lives of people living with HIV/AIDS. The Centre's brief was to produce both academic publications and reports designed to assist government and community groups in the allocation of resources to improve the well-being of people living with HIV/AIDS. Statistical surveys were an important part of our work because governments tend to find that sort of 'hard' data more convincing. However, qualitative research was also essential because, for example, designing effective campaigns to encourage the take up of new medications required a sophisticated understanding of the meanings and interpretations of these drugs for people living with HIV/AIDS. In the mid to late 1990s, the efficacy of treatments for HIV/AIDS was rapidly developing, although many people remained suspicious that the new medications were actually shortening their lives and reducing the quality of life rather than adding anything of benefit.

Our research team conducted a national survey of people living with HIV/AIDS and I noticed a fascinating thing in the survey results: people who identified themselves as religious were less likely to plan for the long term than people who were not religious (Ezzy 2000). This was surprising because I expected religious belief to be associated with greater self-confidence and therefore with greater confidence in the future. I had added the question on religion because of a long-standing academic interest in religious belief.

In a second round of the study we conducted long interviews with people living with HIV/AIDS. The interviews revealed an interesting pattern of responses. People who were not religious were more likely to plan for the long term because they had a greater confidence in medical technology. Secular contemporary society places great trust in science, and that is what these people were doing. In contrast, people who were religious were less confident in the promises of medical technology, probably with some justification given the uncertainty of treatments for HIV/AIDS. However, more interestingly, religious people had changed their orientation towards time.

They celebrated the present, rather than looking forward to gratification in the future (Ezzy 2000). People with a religious world view did have a greater confidence, but that confidence led them to a celebration of the present, and not to a faith in the ability of science to solve the problem of HIV/AIDS. It would have required a very complicated survey to reach that conclusion.

In other words, there are two quite distinct ways of coping with the news that one has HIV and will probably meet an early death. Some people sought certainty in medical science and retained a hope for a long life. Others sought to reframe their lives, celebrating the present. To encourage this latter group to take up new medications would require a quite different campaign to a campaign designed for the former group.

For me, qualitative research is a process of immersing myself in 'the other'. I read existing research carefully, think through how I might understand the problem, and then try to bring these understandings and assumptions into dialogue with the people I am researching. The analysis process begins in the interviews. I always do as many of the interviews as I can myself. I try to listen to what the person is saying, to imagine how they see the world, what matters to them and how they choose what they do. More than that, I try to feel about things as they feel. When I write an academic paper I often 'feel' the argument before I think it, although not always. It is also that way for me with qualitative research – I try to 'feel into' the world of the people I am studying as much as I try to understand it intellectually (Behar 1996).

Once all the interviews were completed I transcribed the first of my interviews and then arranged for the others to be transcribed. I try to transcribe at least one of my interviews. It seems to provide an important opportunity for reflection and to deepen my understanding. Next I read through the interview transcripts. I print out my interviews on the left side of a landscape page and write notes on the right-hand side. As I read and write I also write notes in a book about what seem to be the themes and issues that emerge from each interview. Eventually, I create an index that lists the main themes and the interview and page number where good examples of the themes can be found. From this I write up my results.

Cecilia Orona (1990) describes a methodology of analysing qualitative data that involves long periods of reading, sitting and reflecting. Without this sort of processing time qualitative data analysis becomes mundane, simply a repetition of what we already expect to find. However, when the analyst is prepared to follow the example of Ruth Behar's description of *The Vulnerable Observer* as '*Anthropology that Breaks Your Heart*', we can, perhaps, see beyond our own preconceptions and genuinely allow the voice of the 'other' in our interviews to provide new windows of interpretation and understanding.

It is still a traumatic experience for me to read some of the interview transcripts. I struggled for some time about what to do with the interview with the man with HIV/AIDS who confessed to having unprotected sex in gay venues in Sydney. After discussions with leaders in HIV/AIDS community organisations, I decided that the best course of action was to bring it to the attention of various service providers. There is one interview with a young mother whose child died of AIDS, and who was herself only diagnosed as HIV positive as a consequence of her child's illness. I often have to go for a walk after reading her interview.

Perhaps more confronting was the different understanding of death that some of these people with HIV/AIDS had developed. It led me to ask difficult and sometimes uncomfortable questions about the possibility of my own death. If the possibility of my own death was confronting, it was even more difficult to ask others about the possibility of their death. I never asked it directly, always hinting and suggesting, and often withdrawing when I saw that the person I was interviewing did not want to discuss the topic. However, most of the people I interviewed were very comfortable talking about death. I still remember the interview in which my respondent's face lit up into a gorgeous smile as he realised what I was driving at with my questioning. He looked me in the eye and said: 'Everybody's dying darling.' And so we are.

Behar, R. 1996, *The vulnerable observer: Anthropology that breaks your heart*, Beacon Press, Boston.

Ezzy, D. 2000, 'Illness narratives: Time, hope and HIV', *Social Science and Medicine*, vol. 50, pp. 605–17.

Orona, C. 1990, 'Temporality and identity loss due to Alzheimer's disease', *Social Science and Medicine*, vol. 30, pp. 1247–56.

Recommended reading

Coffey, A. & Atkinson, P. 1996, *Making sense of qualitative data: Complementary research strategies*, Sage Publications, Thousand Oaks, California.

Denzin, N. & Lincoln, Y.S. (eds) 2003, *Collecting and interpreting qualitative materials*, Sage Publications, Thousand Oaks, California.

Gee, J.P. 2005, *An introduction to discourse analysis: Theory and method*, 2nd edn, Routledge, London.

Pryke, M., Rose, G. & Whatmore, S. 2003, *Using social theory: Thinking through research*, Sage Publications in association with the Open University, London.

Silverman, D. 2001, *Interpreting qualitative data: Methods for analysing talk, text and interaction*, 2nd edn, Sage Publications, London.

eight
WRITING QUALITATIVE RESEARCH

Writing serves at least two important roles in qualitative research projects. It is a valuable tool for thinking and part of the analytic process. It is also the most commonly used method of disseminating the results from qualitative research. In Chapter Two I described dissemination as the final stage in the research process. The dissemination of research in written form is important for a range of reasons. It allows other people to read about the research, making it possible for them to learn from the research. This may include learning about research practices and using the results from research to improve practice or develop new research projects (Ueland 1991). Disseminating information about the ways the research was conducted, how the data was analysed, the results and the implications of those results also makes the project available for scrutiny from peers and the wider public. If you remember back to Chapter One of this book, I described research as a public activity. Furthermore, publications arising from research are a widely used measure of success for individual researchers, research teams and for the institutions in which they work or study. At a pragmatic level, it is important to publish from your research, as this will make it easier for you to acquire research funding in the future.

This chapter provides guidance for researchers unfamiliar with presenting qualitative research in a written form. Unlike quantitative research, where researchers can disseminate their results using tables, graphs and numbers, qualitative researchers are largely dependent on the written word. While there are alternative ways of expressing qualitative research, such as through oral presentations, film and photographs, the majority of qualitative research will be presented in written form.

Background to writing in qualitative research

Results from qualitative studies are commonly presented in a detailed narrative. The most common formats for presenting the results from qualitative research are theses, journal articles, books, formal reports and conference papers. However, in some projects researchers may find it more useful to report on their research in the form of newsletters, posters, handouts, community forums and in seminar situations. The main challenge in reporting on qualitative research lies in the necessity for the researcher(s) to convey the complexity and vitality of their research through the medium of the written word. As Marvasti (2004:124) describes it, 'we have to use words to describe other words'.

Another important difference between quantitative and qualitative research is the relative importance of writing to the overall research process. In quantitative research, preparing a written report is seen as the final dissemination stage in the research process. In contrast, for qualitative researchers, writing is also seen as part of data analysis and dissemination. Writing is a 'way of "knowing" – a method of discovery and analysis' (Richardson 2003:499).

> Most fundamentally, analysis is about the representation or reconstruction of social phenomena. We do not simply 'collect' data; we fashion them out of our transactions with other men and women. Likewise we do not merely report what we find; we create accounts of social life, and in doing so we construct versions of the social worlds and social actors we observe. (Coffey & Atkinson 1996:108)

Writing in fact plays a *crucial* role in analysing qualitative data. Coffey and Atkinson describe writing as 'an analytic issue' (1996:117). Whichever approach to analysis a researcher uses, they will inevitably reach a point where they have to transform their results (i.e. a list of themes or descriptions of narratives) into a discussion that is meaningful in terms of their research project and the audience for their work. Personally, I find that the act of 'writing up' increases the sophistication and complexity of my analysis. It often helps me to move from merely describing what I found in my research to attributing certain meanings to these findings, relating these findings to theories and other research and drawing conclusions. Consequently, the act of writing is part of the interpretive process.

Amir Marvasti (2004) provides a wonderful description of the way writing his doctoral dissertation forced him to question his original analysis about the homeless. His research was an ethnographic study, and after interviewing a number of homeless people he had developed a set of propositions about the nature and meaning of being homeless. However, when he started to 'write up' his results, he discovered that his original analysis simply didn't provide him with enough to write about.

> As I put into writing my many ideas and organised my observation into different chapters, I quickly learned that in the process of moving from vague insights to a coherently articulated text many new leads are generated. At the same time, what I had previously thought were ground-breaking ideas turned out to be platitudes. Once I put them into writing, they were much less profound than I originally thought them to be . . . writing in a sense becomes a way of thinking about and analysing data. (Marvasti 2004:120–1)

Other researchers have also spoken about the important role played by writing in qualitative research (Richardson 1990, 2003; Rice & Ezzy 1999; Grbich 1999; Meloy 1994). There are two key issues related to writing that beginner researchers should be aware of. The first is that qualitative researchers need to start writing as soon as possible during their research project. Instead of waiting until they know what they want to say or have results to present, qualitative researchers should view writing as a 'dynamic and creative process' (Richardson 2003:501).

The second is that in a qualitative research project, the researcher shouldn't try to emulate a standard research paper or dissertation from quantitative research. Instead, they need to recognise the unique and valuable characteristics of qualitative research that inevitably mean any written reporting may differ from a standard quantitative research report. At the very least, it will be longer in size and largely descriptive.

Factors to consider when planning your writing

Important factors to consider when writing about your qualitative research project are the intended audience, the methodology of the project, rigour, ethics and the purpose and context of the research. Each of these issues is discussed in detail below.

The audience

The audience for the research has a significant impact on how a researcher will present their results and findings. 'Because each audience has different needs and expectations, a single piece of writing cannot serve all audiences simultaneously' (Rice & Ezzy 1999:237). It follows that results from a single research project may need to be written up in several different ways to suit different audiences. For example, a project conducted by a graduate student may eventually be presented in the form of an academic thesis, several journal articles, a seminar presentation and in a report to a funding body. Each of these will vary in terms of the language used, level of detail required and the overall emphasis (Wolcott 2001).

For example, academic audiences tend to have far more demanding expectations about describing and critiquing methodology and will expect a comprehensive literature review and critical discussion about the project in addition to descriptions of results. In contrast, a report to a funding body will contain less critique and debate but will be more policy- and outcome-orientated (Grbich 1999:259–60). Such a report would also need to include an account detailing the financial costs associated with the project and possibly the results from an evaluation. In contrast, an oral presentation for a seminar is likely to make greater use of visual presentation methods and, for clarity, will often focus on key results or on a single aspect of the study.

Another – and closely associated – issue that impacts on expectations about how best to 'write up' qualitative research is the academic discipline in which the researcher is working. For some researchers, disciplinary expectations about writing up research are relatively straightforward. For example, an anthropologist would be expected to cite anthropological sources and theories and to present their work in a way similar to other anthropologists. This holds true for researchers working within other established academic disciplines – like sociology, geography and education – with a tradition of qualitative research. However, health researchers working within multidisciplinary and applied fields, such as primary care, public health and nursing, and those conducting evaluation, often find it difficult to make decisions about whose work needs to be cited and how to present their data and analysis because they are not working within clear disciplinary parameters. In this case, decisions may need to be made according to the expected audience for their research and the methodology of their project.

Methodology

At some level, a theoretical underpinning of a qualitative research project may have little impact on the writing up. The vast majority of write-ups will follow fairly standard patterns used to report on a research project (more on this later in the chapter). However, because methodology impacts on research questions, the types of data collected and the analysis, there is a relationship between any theoretical perspectives underpinning a project and how the written report will look. This may include the level of detail expected in describing results, the amount and nature of empirical data presented, the form and scope of analytical statements, the structure of work and the expected size of the work. For example, an ethnographic study will usually include considerable detail and discussion about the methods used to gather empirical data and may be characterised by 'thick ethnographic description'. It will also include a lengthy scene-setting discussion that may include historical details and various other types of information (geographic, ecological, medical etc). Consequently, written papers tend to be large, rigorous and comprehensive.

In contrast, research conducted from a postmodern feminist position is unlikely to include detail about sampling methods or data collection techniques. Due to the feminist and postmodern focus on representing multiple voices and perspectives, the data might be presented in innovative and unconventional styles, such as a poem or a play. Instead of the usual report format, the researchers would try to decentre the researcher 'in favour of multivocal and other presentations' (Grbich 1999:276; Lather 1988).

Methodology also impacts on the ways that language is used. This is closely related to the presentation differences mentioned above and the disciplinary background of the research (discussed below). However, the language used will also reflect the theoretical underpinnings of a project due to the associations between writing genres and theories. Examples include the focus on personal narrative accounts in phenomenological projects and the conscious interweaving of 'data and theoretical concepts' found in grounded theory projects (Grbich 1999:263).

However, the association between methodology and language is most apparent in relation to expectations about how the researcher refers to themselves and how they convey the experiences or viewpoints of research participants. It is now commonplace to use personal pronouns in the majority of qualitative writing. This reflects a widespread recognition that a researcher's personal characteristics are an integral aspect of their study and that they will have feelings about the participants and the events they become involved in (Berg 2004). However, projects with methodologies such as grounded theory or traditional ethnography still tend to be written in largely neutral language with little use of emotive or overtly political language (Berg 2004; Kelle 2001; Strauss & Corbin 1990). Many researchers – both quantitative and qualitative alike – recommend that social science maintain a value-neutral position. From this perspective, social scientists are expected to study the world around them as external investigators (Berg 2004:155).

In contrast, researchers working with methodologies derived from certain feminist or postmodern perspectives may choose to use language styles that aim to shock or give a particular and highly personal insight into the thoughts or physical sensations of either the researcher(s) or the research participants (Ronai 1992; Ellis & Bochner 1992).

Rigour

Writing about a research project should reflect any rigour-promoting strategies used in the research project. There is little point in developing a rigorous research design if you neglect to reflect this in your final report. As described in Chapter Three, rigour can be achieved in a number of different ways. At a general level, a rigorous qualitative research project is one with an appropriate methodology, suitable data collection methods, a reflexive and theoretically informed analysis and adherence to high research standards in relation to ethics and the political aspects of the project. All of these factors need to be made visible and be clearly explained and justified in any written reports arising from the project (Cheek 2004; Rice & Ezzy 1999).

Specific strategies to improve the rigour of a research project also require careful consideration when writing about the research. Two such strategies are researcher reflexivity and transparency of methods and analysis. Reflexivity can be reflected in the style of writing and in the content. The researcher can write in such a way that their presence and role in the research is clearly apparent. They could also include sections in the report where they explicitly discuss their role and reflect upon the research and their analysis (Finlay 2002; Marcus 1994). Transparency of methods requires that a researcher carefully explains and justifies their method, including sampling, recruitment, specific data collection methods, data recording, maintenance and storage of data (Silbey 2003; Seale 1999). Transparency of analysis requires that the researcher clearly describes and justifies the analytic strategies used and places these in a theoretical context. It also requires them to present sufficient examples so that a reader can follow the interpretive process and judge the credibility and trustworthiness of the researcher's conclusions for themselves (Lincoln & Guba 1985).

Ethics

A detailed discussion of ethical issues in qualitative research was provided in Chapter Two. Ethical considerations related to a research project should be discussed in the writing and dissemination phase of a research project. This is good research practice; however, in many cases it will also be mandatory. For example, most funding bodies and some peer-reviewed journals expect a researcher to include copies of information sheets for participants, signed consent forms and letters of approval from institutional review boards (ethics committees) with any submissions for publication or final reports.

There may also be ethical issues to consider that are directly related to the written reporting of a project. For example, two important ethical issues are the protection of research participants and the maintenance of confidentiality (Grbich 1999; Lofland & Lofland 1984). When reporting on qualitative research, the identities of research participants should not be disclosed. At a minimum, this will require the use of pseudonyms for people and places; disguising other identifying information, such as work-places and age; or even merging the accounts from several participants into one. It may also be necessary to omit certain examples or details from the written reporting to protect research participants (Marvasti 2004:136). For example, in a study involving interviews with community nurses in three rural towns, where there are only a small number of nurses in each town, any details that allow the location of the towns to be identified could lead to the identification of the research participants.

The research context

In Chapter One I wrote that research does not exist independently. Instead, it is linked in with other people's work. This aspect of the research process becomes apparent when a researcher starts to write about their research. A researcher needs to locate their work in relation to the research and writings of others. This can be thought of as 'framing the research'. When thinking about how your research could be framed, it is useful to consider what you are trying to achieve in your research project. Listed below are three possibilities. Note that, in reality, many research projects fall somewhere in between the following groupings:

1   Investigating a particular situation or research problem, using a theory or pre-existing framework as an orientating framework (e.g. theories of medical dominance, feminist theories, Foucauldian theory or Marxist theory). Your original research questions will have been developed in the light of the theoretical framework; therefore, the project has already been framed by the theory. Your writing should describe and discuss important aspects of this theory or framework and demon-strate how your research and findings relate to it. The writing will also need to reflect a process of moving backwards and forwards between your empirical data and the theory/theories.

2 Exploratory research that could be described as theory-building rather than theory-driven (i.e. hoping to learn something new about a situation that might lead to the development of a set of statements about the phenomena under study). In this type of project, the act of writing will signal a shift towards greater abstraction and generalisation. This reflects a shift in your thinking, away from the individual instances in your data and towards identifying larger patterns, trends, themes and linkages. Many researchers find that they need to use other researchers' theories and ideas during this stage of the analysis; for example, developing some type of theoretically informed schema to describe their findings.

3 Describing a situation or presenting the point of view of research participants. This third situation is common in applied health research. If this fits your project, you will still have a lot of issues to consider. For example, you have most likely been asked to do this research for a reason, so the research findings will need to be related to a bigger research problem or social issue. This will need a degree of extrapolation. Descriptive studies also require considerable reflection about which aspects of the situation the researcher is trying to describe.

Reflecting on the purpose of your research is a useful starting point when attempting to frame your research findings. In addition to giving some guidance about what you are trying to achieve in your writing, it should also help you to identify other written reports to read. Reading other qualitative research articles, books and reports is probably the best way of learning about the options available when presenting your own research.

Qualitative research as a 'good story'

The findings from qualitative research projects are usually greatly interesting; however, books, articles and reports describing this research often go unread because they are written in a boring way (Richardson 2003:501). Richardson advises researchers to try and capture the vivid and creative nature of their research through effective writing practices. This requires a different mindset to reporting on quantitative research. Qualitative researchers need to be able to tell a 'good story'.

> Unlike quantitative work, which can be interpreted through its tables and summaries, qualitative work depends on people reading it. Just as a piece of literature is not equivalent to its 'plot summary', qualitative research is

not contained in its abstracts. Qualitative research has to be read, not scanned; its meaning is in the reading. (Richardson 2003:501)

The storytelling aspect of qualitative research writing is likely to be a challenge for researchers who are only familiar with quantitative research and the relatively dry writing associated with the health sciences. The main difficulties that my students and colleagues experience seem to arise from uncertainty about referring to themselves and their own ideas and experiences, confusion about how to extrapolate and draw conclusions from non-generalisable research, and a disinclination to accept that reporting on qualitative research requires effective storytelling. 'The story-like quality of qualitative research is seen as un-scientific and not objective from the point of view of quantitative researchers' (Rice & Ezzy 1999:245).

Coffey and Atkinson (1996) provide some useful advice in their chapter on writing and representation. They recommend that qualitative researchers reflect on what it takes to write an interesting story. This might involve reading fiction and non-fiction works. They also suggest that researchers take time to consider the different units of narrative they might like to include in their writing. Examples include describing the lives, experiences or views of individuals, shifting to describe an act or event (including recurrent patterns or speech) then discussing groups or populations (Coffey & Atkinson 1996:114–16). To assist with this task, the authors present the following list, adapted from Spradley (1970:210–11). The list outlines six levels of statement, moving from the general to the particular, which when used together make for effective writing. Coffey and Atkinson suggest that reflecting on these different levels of generality constitutes good analytic discipline and should facilitate interesting and effective writing about qualitative research.

Level 1
Universal statements: all-encompassing writing about social actors, their behaviour, culture or environmental situation.
Level 2
Cross-cultural descriptive statements: statements about two or more societies, including assertions that are true for some but not necessarily all societies.
Level 3
General statements about a society or cultural group: statements that combine generality with specificity, making some general points about a particular group.

Level 4

General statements about a specific cultural scene: statements, still of a general nature, that capture some of the themes of a particular social scene.

Level 5

Specific statements about a cultural domain: statements about how social actors use linguistic devices and folk terms to describe events, objects and activities.

Level 6

Specific incident statements: writing that takes the reader immediately to a particular behaviour or particular events, demonstrating cultural knowledge in action.

(Coffey & Atkinson 1996:114)

Richardson (2003) also recommends the use of specific writing exercises to improve writing about qualitative research. She emphasises the importance of demystifying writing, nurturing the researcher's voice, and 'serving the process of discovery' through writing (2003:527). Among a long list of recommendations Richardson suggests the following: avoid using old worn-out metaphors; search out excellent examples of qualitative research writing and spend time thinking about how the paper was written; join or start a writing group; use field notes as an opportunity to 'expand your writing vocabulary'; keep a journal about your research and writing; experiment with less conventional writing styles and ways of presenting qualitative research (2003:529–30).

Common writing structures and styles

The vast majority of reports, theses and journal articles follow a similar format to the one described in Chapter Two in the section on developing a research plan. The major difference is that a research plan describes how data collection and analysis will occur. In contrast, the final report, thesis or article is able to include the results from the data collection and analysis. Accordingly, this section of a final report tends to be much larger and more important than in a research plan. Because of this similarity, revisiting your research plan is often a useful way to get started when writing up a project. It will form the bones of the standard qualitative writing plan.

Standard writing plan

Several key components are present in almost all qualitative research papers, reports and theses (Marvasti 2004:126; Rice & Ezzy 1999:239). These are an introduction, literature review, methods, analysis and results and conclusion. The introduction section enables the writer to briefly outline the research problem and research questions and to explain the purpose of the research. The literature review should consist of a critical discussion about previous research on the topic. The literature reviewed should be current and relevant. The discussion should be presented in such a way as to explain 'why and how the research problem came to be defined in this particular way' (Grbich 1999:260). Literature reviews may also include a discussion about the theoretical perspectives underpinning the research design (methodology). However, this is often addressed in the methods section. The methods section is often quite detailed and should include information about the sample, data collection, ethics and the methods of analysis used. The analysis section is akin to the results section in a quantitative research paper. When reporting the findings from a qualitative research project, it is important to 'draw clear, logical connections between the empirical data and your interpretations' (Marvasti 2004:127). It is also important to support your analysis with examples from the data. Some researchers like to interweave their analysis with discussion about other studies and the wider literature. However, this can also be done in the discussion section. The discussion section is a place to draw together the various elements of the project. This often involves providing a brief overview of the project, extrapolating from the analysis to discuss the implications of the results and reflecting on the study design. Many researchers like to discuss how the study could be improved and to make suggestions for future studies in the area.

Themes, narratives and stories

Some researchers attempt to reflect their findings and analysis in the structure of the written report. For instance, in a study where the analysis produced a number of large overarching themes, the names of these themes could be used as subheadings to organise the analysis section. In Joan Sayre's (2000) paper about how patients explain their mental illness, she uses the six attribution categories that emerged from a grounded theory analysis to structure the presentation of results. Therefore in the analysis section each subheading represents a theme. The themes are problem, disease, crisis, punishment, ordination and violation.

Under each subheading, she describes the nature of patient accounts grouped under this theme and provides examples and contextual data.

Alternatively, a researcher investigating narratives is unlikely to structure the analysis section of a report or article using themes. Instead, they may prefer to use organising devices derived from narrative analysis. For example, Bailey (2004) investigated narratives in accounts of acute exacerbations given by people living with chronic obstructive pulmonary disease. The style of narrative analysis used by Bailey required her to identify types of story and then to systematically analyse these by parsing them into identified story elements, such as abstract, orientation and compelling action. Subsequently, she identified 'story events and meanings from the story elements' (2004:763). In a journal article reporting her results, Bailey focused on vulnerability stories as these were the most frequently told stories in the interviews. When presenting these results, Bailey defined what she meant by the term 'vulnerability stories' and then organised her analysis using the following subheadings: story structure and content, meaning of emotional vulnerability stories, visibility functions of emotional vulnerability stories, and the legitimisation of emotional vulnerability stories. She then illustrated her analysis with a comprehensive case example that included large sections of interview transcript.

The narrative aspect of qualitative research can also be expressed in written form through the use of less structured presentation and writing styles. These are well suited to phenomenological and ethnographic projects; however, they can be used to improve the storytelling aspect of any qualitative research report. Grbich (1999) lists vignettes, anecdotes, layers of information, pastiche, quotes of larger sections of interview data and ethnographic description as useful ways of expressing the meaning and content of qualitative research. Two of these that I have found to be particularly enjoyable and useful are vignettes and thick ethnographic description. Thick ethnographic description is a variation in descriptive writing. Grbich (1999:269) contrasts the thin description often used in research writing with thick description by using the following examples:

Thin description: 'Jane went into labour at 7.30am. By 9am her contractions were coming every five minutes so they set off to hospital. Jane was delivered of a baby girl at 10.45am.'

Thick ethnographic description: 'Jane woke at seven o'clock. Her stomach felt uncomfortable, and labour started half an hour later. She woke Jim, who reassured her that there was no rush, that he and Jill (their two-year-old) needed breakfast before embarking on the trip to the city. Jane did not eat but half-sat, half-lay on a bean bag . . .' (Grbich 1999:269)

Vignettes are compressed stories 'narrating what the researcher has learned over a period' (1999:267). Vignettes can be used to convey case studies, to give a feeling for a particular situation, setting or aspect of the research. I often use vignettes to set a scene before using quotations as examples. Thus before using a quote, I provide a small vignette to place the quote, research setting or research participant in context. See the following example from my PhD thesis (Hansen 2001):

> Another pattern which frequently occurred when doctors were talking about uncertainty and the causes of disease was that their talk about uncertainty related to explaining disease, however phrased, was usually followed by a more up-beat and positive discussion where issues such as the value of medical research or the importance of lifestyle modification as a way of preventing disease were emphasised. This pattern is apparent in the following example:
>
> Emily: But do you ever have a patient who *has* been working really hard to take care of themselves for a long time but still gets seriously ill? How do you make sense of that?
>
> Dr J: (emphatically) Yep. Yes, that happens quite frequently. There is no answer for that. All I can tell them is that I just don't know.
>
> Emily: Is that difficult for you as a doctor to do?
>
> Dr J: Yes, it is. Because it makes you realise yourself how vulnerable you are. And that is what it really comes down to. We are all vulnerable. (she pauses) But one of the things that I really enjoy about medicine is empowering people. The old style medicine was that we don't tell them anything. I don't like that approach and I never have done. To me it has always been 'what can I tell the person that they couldn't find out for themselves and that will help them to look after themself?'.

Mixed methods studies

Creswell (2003:222) suggest three different ways to structure reports for multi-method projects depending on the study design. Sequential studies are characterised by two phases of data collection and analysis, one qualitative and one quantitative. These phases occur in sequence. For example, an exploratory qualitative phase is followed by a quantitative phase. In reports for this type of study design, the writer 'typically will present the project as two distinct phases, with separate headings for each phase' (2003:222). In the discussion section, they comment on the two types of research and explain how they extend or elaborate the other.

Concurrent studies are akin to the complementary research designs described in Chapter One. Data collection and analysis are likely to occur concurrently, and the results from the qualitative and quantitative aspects of the research are compared for convergence or to develop a fuller picture of the issue under study. In this type of design, the analysis and interpretation of qualitative and quantitative research may be presented in a combined form. 'The structure of this type of mixed methods study does not clearly make a distinction between the quantitative and qualitative phases' (Creswell 2003:222). I was involved in a mixed methods study investigating the diagnosis and management of chronic obstructive pulmonary disease in general practice. We collected quantitative data from an audit of patient case notes, medical tests and questionnaires. We also collected qualitative data from interviews and focus groups with patients and GPs. Our research team presented overviews of all of the data in conference presentations (Walters et al. 2005; Hansen et al. 2004). However, we decided to present different aspects of the data in a number of journal articles. One of these used a selection of quantitative data and qualitative data but focused on only one issue – barriers to the use of spirometry in general practice (Walters et al. 2005). This article discussed results from focus groups with GPs and our audit of patient case notes. We are currently writing two additional articles: one discusses data from health-related quality-of-life questionnaires completed by patients and semi-structured interviews with patients. This article will be sent to a medical journal. The other is focused entirely on interview data from patients and discusses this data using existing sociological theories about the ways in which people explain the causes of their chronic illness. It will be sent to a sociological journal.

Creswell describes the third type of mixed methods study as transformative. By this term he is referring to research conducted using a Participatory Action framework and therefore 'typically involving the advocacy issue in the beginning of the study and then using either the sequential or concurrent structure as a means of organising the content of the study' (Creswell 2003:222). The reports for this type of study would be organised similarly to the structures described above, with the addition of a separate section focused on advancing change or reform as a result of the study.

In relation to publication in journals, many researchers choose to report different aspects of their study in the form of individual articles. This is often necessary because of the word limits imposed by the majority of academic journals. For example, Wager et al. (2004) conducted a large study involving a cost-benefit of a post-partum infant home-visit program in South Carolina. Their study used quantitative and qualitative methods (Bradford et al. 2002). While the report from the study described results from both research approaches, the authors chose to write an article reporting only the qualitative results from focus groups with mothers. Their article was published in the journal, *Public Health Nursing*.

Reports

Most applied research, including evaluations, will be presented in a report format. Funding bodies also require reports at the conclusion of a project. Reports are often used when making decisions and changes related to a project, organisation or policy.

Reports usually follow the standard structure described above (introduction, literature review, methods, analysis, discussion) with the addition of an executive summary and lists of recommendations. An executive summary 'presents the essential elements of the report from the introduction through to the recommendations and outcomes' (Manser et al. 2004:2).

I have often found it helpful to look at other reports written for the organisation to get a feel for their expectations about formatting. Reports should adhere to expectations about scholarly writing, with full reference lists and a discussion about methodology. Transparency and inclusiveness are overarching principles that can be used to guide decisions about the framework for a report and decisions about what to report, the quality of report (Global Reporting Initiative 2002).

Journal articles

Getting results from research published in the form of articles in peer-reviewed journals is important for dissemination and as a measure of success for researchers. Unlike most reports, journal articles are widely distributed and available for searching using on-line databases and library catalogues (Morse 1994).

Most journals have strict guidelines about the size and structure for their articles. It follows that any researchers planning to write their results in the form of a journal article need to select an appropriate journal and obtain a copy of their instructions for authors. Appropriate journals include those that have already published articles from projects with similar methodologies and methods or issues or problems; journals with a readership suited to the research project; and journals that are well recognised and respected in your field or profession. Qualitative health research has been successfully published in mainstream medical, nursing and allied health journals and in sociological, anthropological, public health and qualitative research journals. There are also a number of journals devoted solely to qualitative research.

The size restrictions posed by many journals tend to create a challenge when writing about qualitative research. This is particularly apparent in health-related journals, as these frequently have tight restrictions on word length. In contrast, sociological, anthropological and qualitative research specific journals will often accept quite lengthy articles – up to 8000 words.

Useful strategies for adapting research findings for a journal article include focusing on one or two aspects of the research and using visual display techniques, such as tables and charts. As previously mentioned, researchers often publish several different articles from a single project, each focused on a different issue or aspect of the research (Richardson 2003; Rice & Ezzy 1999).

Theses

Qualitative research conducted as part of a graduate or postgraduate degree is likely to be reported on in the form of a thesis. Academic qualitative research offers a researcher a broad range of possibilities in terms of research design and presentation styles. The examiners of the thesis will be skilled and experienced researchers with a wide breadth of knowledge. As such they are likely to be aware of the less common presentation and writing styles available to qualitative researchers; for example, auto-ethnography and postmodern and feminist narratives (Grbich 1999:263).

Theses tend, however, to follow the standard format for presenting research outlined above. They often present an argument or put forward a particular point of view and the literature review may include considerable critique of other theories and research. Theses also need to include considerable detail about the methodology, ethics and the strengths and weaknesses of the research method.

Because theses are assessed, a student should take guidance from their research supervisors about the best ways to structure them and the style of writing to be used. It is also useful to read other theses from your area to pick up ideas about the different ways they can be structured and possible writing styles.

Final writing tips

As you can see, there are many issues to consider when writing up your research, making it difficult to give any hard and fast rules for how written descriptions and discussions arising from qualitative research should look. The best way to find out in relation to your own research is to read examples of previously published qualitative research in your area. In addition, your supervisors, peers and colleagues may all have useful advice. Advice and feedback from others is particularly important in the early stages when you have just started writing and then again in the later stages, such as editing and formatting. All experienced writers know the value of getting feedback on their writing.

The following checklist is applicable to most qualitative research reports, theses, articles and so on. Following these suggestions should greatly improve the quality of any written or oral presentation of qualitative research findings.

Be reflexive

Think critically about your own ideas and assumptions and those of other people. Question your analysis. Include evidence of this critical thinking in your write-up.

Be verifiable

The reader should be able to reach their own conclusions about the 'truth' of your analysis. The best way for them to do this is for them to read sufficient examples from your data and for you to describe how you reached your conclusions. Don't hide your tracks. Clearly explain your methods of data collection and analysis.

Be accountable

You are responsible for your analysis. It may have 'real world' impact. Don't hide, be present. I like to know who a researcher is when I read their work. I like to know why they did the research and their relationship to the 'researched'.

Be ethical

Adhere to guidelines for ethical conduct in research. When writing up your research, respect your participants and ensure their confidentiality. At times, this may mean leaving out excerpts of interviews, even if they are really interesting. Most professional organisations and academic institutions have an ethics committee or at least a statement about ethical research. Use them.

Stay focused around the research problem/research questions

These will ground you if you feel like you have too much data and don't know what to include in your write-up. Remember, it is often possible to write up more than one report from your research.

Remember your audience

How you present your data, the language you use, the level of detail etc will be contingent on your audience. Equally, there are differences between a government report, community feedback, an internal report for your organisation etc.

Be professional in terms of your background/academic discipline
Meet the standards expected, reference correctly, use reputable sources, conduct a literature review that utilises sources from a range of backgrounds rather than just using whatever is lying around the office, and confer with colleagues for advice, suggestions.

Chapter summary

This chapter provided guidance for researchers unfamiliar with presenting qualitative research in a written form. It began with a discussion about the background to qualitative research writing. The importance of writing to qualitative data analysis and dissemination was emphasised. Next to be raised were issues to consider when planning what to write about and how to do so. These issues were the audience, methodology, rigour, ethics and the context of the research project. Then I discussed the storytelling aspects of qualitative research and the importance of striving to 'tell a good story' when writing about your research. The next section of the chapter described the writing structures and styles commonly used by qualitative researchers. The chapter closed with some final tips for 'good' writing about qualitative research provided in the form of a checklist.

Recommended reading

Becker, H.S. 1986, *Writing for social scientists: How to finish your thesis, book or article*, University of Chicago Press.

Behar, R. & Gordon, D.A. (eds) 1995, *Women writing culture*, University of California Press, Berkeley.

Ellis, C. & Bochner A.P. (eds) 1996, *Composing ethnography: Alternative forms of qualitative writing*, Walnut Creek, AltaMira, California.

Johnstone, M.J. 2004, *Effective writing for health professionals: A practical guide to getting published*, Allen & Unwin, Sydney.

Richardson, L. 1990, *Writing strategies: Reaching diverse audiences*, Sage Publications, Thousand Oaks, California.

Wolcott, H.F. 2001, *Writing up qualitative research*, 2nd edn, Sage Publications, Thousand Oaks, California.

GLOSSARY

Audit trail: The documenting of sampling, methods and analysis to allow others to follow the researcher's thinking and conclusions about the data.

Action Research: See Participatory Action Research.

Active interviewing: Active interviews (a term coined by Holstein & Gubrium 1995) are seen as social occasions where the interviewer and the interviewee jointly create social reality through interaction.

Analysis: The process by which qualitative researchers transform raw empirical data into results, interpretations, conclusions, hypotheses and propositions.

Anonymity: If data is anonymous, the researcher does not know the identities of research participants.

Confidentiality: To maintain the confidentiality of research participants, researchers ensure they cannot be identified in results or written reports. Participants are instructed to maintain the confidentiality of others involved in the study.

Content analysis: Qualitative data is analysed using a system of coding and counting.

Data saturation: A point at which the researcher will cease data collection because the information arising from data becomes repetitive and contains no new ideas. At this point a researcher can be reasonably confident that the inclusion of additional participants is unlikely to produce new ideas.

Deductive reasoning: A process of developing specific predictions (hypotheses) from general principles. This type of reasoning moves from the general to the particular.

Discourse: Dynamic historically and socially situated sets of language and practices through which meaning is produced, reproduced and transformed. Examples are discourses on childbirth or discourses on diet and heart disease.

Dramaturgy: A dramaturgical approach, both in sociology and else-where, treats everyday behaviour as a theatrical performance. In the social sciences, dramaturgy is strongly associated with the work of Erving Goffman.

Emic perspective (emic view): Insider's, or native's, view of his or her world (*see also* etic perspective).

Ethnography: A research methodology associated with anthropology and sociology that systematically describes the culture of a group of people.

Etic perspective (etic view): Outsider's view of the experiences of a specific cultural group (*see also* emic perspective).

Ethnomethodology: The study of 'ethnomethods', or 'member's methods', derives from a collection of investigations conducted by University of California, Los Angeles, sociologist Harold Garfinkel in the 1950s and '60s.

Field: The research setting. A term often used in ethnographic research.

Field notes: Notes taken by a researcher to record incidents, observations and contextual information.

Focus group: Group discussion on a focused topic.

Hypothesis: A statement that predicts the relationship between variables – specifically, the relationship between the independent and dependent variables.

In-depth interview: See unstructured in-depth interviews.

Informal interview: This type of interview occurs spontaneously, often during participant observation.

Inductive reasoning: A process of reasoning used to develop more general rules from specific observations; this type of reasoning moves from the specific to the more generalised.

Informed consent: Voluntary participation in research by individuals based on a full understanding of the possible benefits and risks.

Interpretivist paradigm: Also called constructivist and naturalistic paradigm. This paradigm assumes that there are multiple interpreta-tions of reality and that the goal of researchers working within this perspective is to understand how individuals construct their own reality within their social context.

Linguistic turn in sociology: During the past two decades, the 'linguistic', or 'rhetorical', turn has emerged as an important intellectual movement in the human and social sciences. Its major implication is that society can be viewed as a text and that social and cultural reality, and the sciences themselves, are linguistic constructions.

Methodology: The justification given for why particular methods of data collection and analysis have been selected. Methodologies are often based on theoretical perspectives or approaches.

Methods: Research techniques for data collection and analysis.

Narrative analysis: An approach to analysing qualitative data that focuses on the structure and nature of narratives, or stories.

Observation: A method of data collection in which data is gathered through visual observations.

Participant: The terms 'research participant', or 'informant', are used in qualitative research as an alternative to the traditional term 'research subject'.

Participatory Action Research (PAR): An approach to qualitative research orientated towards participation action, change and empowerment. The participants become the researchers and vice versa.

Phenomenology: A philosophical school of thought that attempts to describe how the constitution of reality in the acts of our consciousness occurs. Phenomenology focuses on basic processes bestowing meaning on the human world, and its results are significant for those crucial questions of social theory, asking how 'individuals' construct and interpret their reality and how they define situations to give orientation to their actions.

Positivism: In its most general sense, positivism is a doctrine that maintains that the study of the human, or social, world should be organised according to the same principles as the study of the physical, or natural, world.

Postmodernism: A set of intellectual propositions that challenge the assumptions embedded within modern thought. Emphasis is placed on the plural nature of reality, multiple voices, multiple views of reality, and an interest in representation.

Poststructuralism: Associated with postmodernism but characterised by a focus on the 'exploration and analysis of texts' (Cheek 2001:6).

Purposive sampling: Also called purposeful sampling. A non-probability sampling strategy in which the researcher selects participants who are considered to be the most appropriate for a qualitative study.

Reification: A concept based on the idea that people create their social worlds, especially larger social structures and institutions. However, over time, people come to lose sight of this fact. Instead these structures and institutions come to be seen by people as 'things' that exist independently of the people who created them.

Reflexivity: 'An acknowledgement of the role and influence of the researcher on the research project' (Rice & Ezzy 1999:257).

'Rich' data: 'A wide and diverse range of information collected over a relatively prolonged period of time' (Lofland & Lofland 1984:11). A term associated with ethnographic and naturalistic research.

Research question: A clear statement, in the form of a question, used to guide a research project.

Research problem: An issue that lends itself to systematic investigation through research.

Rigour: Traditional measures of scientific rigour are objectivity, reliability and validity. These are unsuited to qualitative research. Thus alternative criteria for rigour have been developed by qualitative researchers. These include credibility, dependability and transferability.

Semi-structured interviews: Where the researcher uses a loose interview guide and asks open-ended questions.

Structured interviews: Where the interviewer asks each respondent the same questions, using a structured interview schedule with closed response categories.

Theme: A recurring issue that emerges during the analysis of qualitative data.

Thematic analysis: An iterative approach aimed at identifying themes in qualitative data.

Theoretical framework: The conceptual underpinning of a research study.

Theory: In its most general sense, a theory describes or explains something. Often it is the answer to 'what', 'when', 'how' or 'why' questions.

Triangulation: Using multiple methods, researchers, theories or data sources for the purpose of confirmation or validation.

Trustworthiness: A term used to describe whether qualitative research has been conducted in such a way that it gives the reader confidence in the findings.

Unstructured in-depth interviews: Interviews conducted without any set research questions.

REFERENCES

Adams, J., Schaffer, A., Lewin, S., Zwarenstein, M. & van der Walt, H. 2003, 'Health systems research training enhances workplace research skills: A qualitative evaluation', *Journal of Continuing Education in the Health Professions*, vol. 23, no. 4, pp. 210–20.

Adib Hagbaghery, M., Salsali, M. & Ahmadi, F. 2004, 'A qualitative study of Iranian nurses' understanding and experiences of professional power', *Human Resources and Health*, vol. 2, no. 1, p. 9.

Adler, P. & Adler, P. 1987, *Membership roles in field research*, Sage Publications, Newbury Park, California.

Albert, E., Hansen, E. & Cook, C. 2003, 'Grass roots research: How to have a stab at your first project and succeed', *Australian Family Physician*, vol. 32, no. 7, pp. 564–7.

Alderson, P. 1998, 'Theories in health care and research: The importance of theories of health care', *British Medical Journal*, vol. 317, pp. 1007–10.

Allen, J. 2003, 'A question of language' in *Using social theory: Thinking through research*, eds M. Pryke, G. Rose & S. Whatmore, Sage Publications, London.

Aljunid, S. 1996, 'How to do (or not to do). Computer analysis of qualitative data: The use of ethnograph', *Health Policy and Planning*, vol. 11, no. 1, pp. 107–11.

Altheide, D. & Johnson, J. 1994, 'Criteria for assessing interpretive validity in qualitative research', in *Handbook of qualitative research*, eds N. Denzin & Y. Lincoln, Sage Publications, Thousand Oaks, California.

Appleton, T.V. 1995, 'Analyzing qualitative interview data – Addressing issues of validity and reliability', *Journal of Advanced Nursing*, vol. 22, no. 5, pp. 993–7.

Armstrong, D., Gosling, A., Weinman, J. & Marteau, T. 1997, 'The place of inter-rater reliability in qualitative research: An empirical study', *Sociology*, vol. 31, pp. 597–606.

Ashmore, M. & Reed, D. 2000, *Innocence and nostalgia in conversation analysis: The dynamic relations of tape and transcript*, available at: http://qualitativeresearch. net/fqs/fqs-eng.htm.

Atkinson, P. 1995, *Medical talk and medical work*, Sage Publications, London.

Atkinson, P. 1997, 'Narrative turn or blind alley?', *Qualitative Health Research*, vol. 7, pp. 325–44.

Atkinson, P. & Silverman, D. 1997, 'Kundera's immorality: The interview society and the invention of self', *Qualitative Inquiry*, vol. 3, no. 3, pp. 324–45.

Australian Health Ethics Committee (1995), *Assessment of qualitative research: Information for institutional ethics committees*.

Avdi, E., Griffin, C. & Brough, S. 2000, 'Patients' constructions of professional knowledge, expertise and authority during assessment and diagnosis of their child for an autistic spectrum disorder', *British Journal of Medical Psychology*, vol. 73, no. part III, pp. 327–38.

Bailey, C.A. 1996, *A guide to field research*, Pine Forge Press, California.

Bailey, P.H. 2001, 'Death stories: Acute exacerbations of chronic obstructive pulmonary disease', *Qualitative Health Research*, vol. 11, pp. 322–38.

Bailey, P.H. 2004, 'The dyspnea-anxiety-dyspnea cycle – COPD patients' stories of breathlessness: "It's scary when you can't breathe"', *Qualitative Health Research*, vol. 14, no. 6, pp. 760–78.

Baker, R. & Hinton, R. 1999, 'Do focus groups facilitate meaningful participation in social research?' in *Developing focus group research: Politics, theory and practice*, R. Barbour & J. Kitzinger (eds), Sage Publications, London.

Baker, T.L. 1994, *Doing social research*, 2nd edn, McGraw-Hill, New York.

Barbour, R. 2001, 'Checklists for improving rigour in qualitative research: A case of the tail wagging the dog?' *British Medical Journal*, vol. 322, pp. 1115–17.

Barbour, R. & Kitzinger, J. 1999, *Developing focus group research: Politics, theory and practice*, Sage Publications, London.

Basch, C.E. 1987, 'Focus group interview: An underutilized research technique for improving theory and practice in health education', *Health Education Quarterly*, vol. 14, no. 4, pp. 411–48.

Bates, B.R., Lynch, J.A., Bevan, J.L. & Condit, C.M. 2004, 'Warranted concerns, warranted outlooks: A focus group study of public understandings of genetic research', *Social Science and Medicine*, vol. 60, no. 2, pp. 331–44.

Baum, F. 1992, Deconstructing the qualitative–quantitative divide in health research, paper presented to Methodological Issues in Qualitative Research Conference, Deakin University, Geelong, Friday 27 November.

Baum, F. 1995, 'Researching public health: Behind the qualitative-quantitative methodological debate', *Social Science and Medicine*, vol. 40, pp. 459–68.

Becker, C. 1992, *Living and relating: An introduction to phenomenology*, Sage Publications, Newbury Park, California.

Becker, H.S. 1986, *Writing for social scientists: How to finish your thesis, book or article*, University of Chicago Press.

Begley, C.M. 1996, 'Using triangulation in nursing research', *Journal of Advanced Nursing*, vol. 24, no. 1, pp. 122–8.

Behar, R. & Gordon, D.A. 1995, *Women writing culture*, University of California Press, Berkeley.

Berg, B.L. 2004, *Qualitative research methods for the social sciences*, Pearson, Boston.

Blaikie, N.W.H. 1991, 'A critique of the use of traingulation in social research', *Quality and Quantity*, vol. 25, no. 2, pp. 115–36.

Blaikie, N.W.H. 1993, *Approaches to social enquiry*, Polity Press, Cambridge.

Bloor, M. 1976, 'Bishop Berkeley and the adenotonsillectomy enigma: An exploration of the social construction of medical disposals', *Sociology*, vol. 10, pp. 43–61.

Blumer, H. 1969, *Symbolic interactionism*, Prentice Hall, Englewood Cliffs.

Borone, T. 2001, *Touching eternity: The enduring outcomes of teaching*, Teachers College Press, New York.

Borreani, C., Miccinesi, G., Brunelli, C. & Lina, M. 2004, 'An increasing number of qualitative research papers in oncology and palliative care: Does it mean a thorough development of the methodology of research?' *Health and Quality of Life Outcomes*, vol. 2, no. 1, p. 7.

Bradford, W.D., Lee, F.W., Jones, W., Kilpatrick, A.O. & Waher, K.A. 2002, *South Carolina Medicaid postpartum/infant home visit program outcome evaluation*. Report to the South Carolina Department of Health and Human Services.

Brannen, J. (ed.) 1992, *Mixing methods: Qualitative and quantitative research*, Avebury, Aldershott.

Brett, J.A., Heimendinger, J., Boender, C., Morin, C. & Marshall, J.A. 2002, 'Using ethnography to improve intervention design', *American Journal of Health Promotion*, vol. 16, no. 6, pp. 331–40.

Britten, N. 1997, 'Qualitative interviews in health research', in *Qualitative research in health care*, eds C. Pope & N. Mays, British Medical Journal (BMJ) Books, London.

Bruner, J. 1990, *Acts of meaning*, Harvard University Press, Cambridge, Massachusetts.

Bruner, J. 1991, 'The narrative construction of reality', *Critical Inquiry*, vol. 18, pp. 1–21.

Burgess, R.G. 1991, 'Keeping field notes' in *Field research: A sourcebook and field manual*, ed. R.G. Burgess, Routledge, New York.

Burgess, R.G. 1993, *Research methods*, Nelson, London.

Burman, E. & Parker, I. (eds) 1993a, *Discourse analytic research*, Routledge, London.

Burman, E. & Parker, I. 1993b, 'Introduction – discourse analysis: The turn to text', in *Discourse analytic research*, eds E. Burman & I. Parker, Routledge, London, pp. 1–16.

Burnard, P. 1991, 'A method of analysing interview transcripts in qualitative research', *Nurse Education Today*, vol. 11, pp. 461–6.

Caracelli, V.J. & Greene, J.C. 1993, 'Data analysis strategies for mixed-method evaluation designs', *Educational Evaluation and Policy Analysis*, vol. 15, pp. 195–207.

Caroleo, O. 2001, 'An ethnographic study examining the impact of a therapeutic recreation program on people with AIDS: In their own words', *Therapeutic Recreation Journal*, vol. 35, no. 2, pp. 155–69.

Carspecken, P.F. 1996, *Critical ethnography in educational research: A theoretical and practical guide*, Routledge, New York.

Casebeer, A.L. & Verhoef, M.J. 1997, 'Combining qualitative and quantitative research methods: Considering the possibilities for enhancing the study of chronic diseases', *Chronic Disease in Canada*, vol. 18, pp. 130–5.

Chang, L.C., Li, I.C. & Liu, C.H. 2004, 'A study of the empowerment process for cancer patients using Freire's dialogical interviewing', *Journal of Nursing Research*, vol. 12, no. 1, pp. 41–50.

Chapman, S. & Lupton, D. 1994, 'Moral tales and medical marvels: Health and medical stories in a week of Australian television', *Media Information Australia*, vol. 72, pp. 94–103.

Charmaz, K. 1983, 'The grounded theory method: An explication and interpretation' in *Contemporary field research*, ed. R. Emerson, Little Brown, Boston.

Charmaz, K. 1990, 'Discovering chronic illness: Using grounded theory', *Social Science and Medicine*, vol. 30, no. 10, pp. 1161–72.

Charmaz, K. 1991, *Good days, bad days: The self in chronic illness and time*, Rutgers University Press, New Brunswick.

Cheek, J. 2000, *Postmodern and poststructural approaches to nursing research*, Sage Publications, Thousand Oaks, California.

Cheek, J. 2004, 'At the margins? Discourse analysis and qualitative research', *Qualitative Health Research*, vol. 14, no. 8, pp. 1140–50.

Cheek, J. & Rudge, T. 1994, 'Inquiry into nursing as a textually mediated discourse', in *Advances in methods of inquiry for nursing*, ed. P. Chinn, Gaithersburg, Aspen, pp. 59–67.

Cheek, J., Shoebridge, J., Willis, E. & Zadoroznyj, M. 1996, *Society and health: Social theory for health workers*, Longman Cheshire, Melbourne.

Cheung, J. & Hocking, P. 2004 'The experience of spousal carers of people with Multiple Sclerosis', *Qualitative Health Research*, vol. 14, no. 2, pp. 153–66.

Chiseri-Strater, E. & Sunstein, B.S. 2001, *Fieldworking: Reading and writing research*, 2nd edn, St Martins Press, New York.

Chui, L. & Knight, D. 1999, 'How useful are focus groups for obtaining the views of minority groups?' in *Developing focus group research: Politics, theory and practice*, eds R. Barbour & J. Kitzinger, Sage Publications, London, pp. 99–112.

Chung, D. & Abbot, D. 1994, '*What is research?*', South Australian Community Health Research Unit, Adelaide.

Clandinin, D.J. & Connelly, F.M. 1999, *Narrative inquiry: Experience and story in qualitative research*, Jossey-Bass, San Fransisco.

Clark, P. & Bowling, A. 1990, 'Quality of everyday life in long stay institutions for the elderly: An observational study of long stay hospital and nursing home care', *Social Science and Medicine*, vol. 30, no. 11, pp. 1201–10.

Clarke, J., Fletcher, P.C. & Schneider, M.A. 2002, 'Mothers caring for children with cancer', *Centres of Excellence for Women's Health Research Bulletin*, vol. 3, no. 1, pp. 6–8.

Cloherty, M., Alexander, J. & Holloway, I. 2004, 'Supplementing breast-fed babies in the UK to protect their mothers from tiredness or distress', *Midwifery*, vol. 20, no. 2, pp. 194–204.

Clough, P. 1994, *Feminist thought*, Blackwell, Oxford.

Coffey, A. & Atkinson, P. 1996, *Making sense of qualitative data: Complementary research strategies*, Sage Publications, Thousand Oaks, California.

Cohen, A.B., Greenwood, D.J. & Harkavay, I. 1992, 'Social research for social change: Varieties of participatory action research', *Collaborative Inquiry*, vol. 7, pp. 2–8.

Cook, M. 1992, 'Computer analyses of qualitative data: A literature review of current issues', *The Australian Journal of Advanced Nursing*, vol. 10, no. 1, pp. 10–3.

Corbin, J. & Morse, J.M. 2003, 'The unstructured interactive interview: Issues of reciprocity and risks when dealing with sensitive topics', *Qualitative Inquiry*, vol. 9, no. 3, pp. 335–54.

Corbin, J. & Strauss, A. 1985, 'Managing chronic illness at home: Three lines of work', *Qualitative Sociology*, vol. 8, no. 3, pp. 224–47.

Corbin, J. & Strauss, A. 1990, 'Grounded theory research: Procedures, canons, and evaluative criteria', *Qualitative Sociology*, vol. 13, no. 1, pp. 3–21.

Corin, E. & Lauzon, G. 1992, 'Positive withdrawal and the quest for meaning: The reconstruction of experience among schizophrenics', *Psychiatry, Interpersonal and Biological Processes*, vol. 55, no. 3, pp. 266–79.

Cornford, C.S., Harley, J. & Oswald, N. 2004, 'The "2-week rule" for suspected breast carcinoma: A qualitative study of the views of patients and professionals', *British Journal of General Practice*, vol. 54, no. 505, pp. 584–8.

Counterbalance Foundation Online Glossary, definition of postmodernism, accessed 18 April 2005 http://www.pbs.org/faithandreason/gengloss/postm-body.html.

Creswell, J.W. 2003, *Research design: Qualitative, quantitative and mixed methods approaches*, Sage Publications, Thousand Oaks, California.

Crick, M. 1989, 'Shifting identities in the research process: An essay in personal anthropology', in *Doing fieldwork: Eight personal accounts of social research*, ed. J. Perry, Deakin University Printery, Geelong, pp. 24–40.

Cutliffe, J.R. & Ramcharan, P. 2002, 'Leveling the playing field? Exploring the merits of the ethics-as-process approach for judging qualitative research proposals', *Qualitative Health Research*, vol. 12, no. 7, pp. 1000–10.

Daly, J. & McDonald, I. 1992 'Covering your back: Strategies for qualitative research in clinical settings', *Qualitative Health Research*, vol. 2, no. 4, pp. 416–38.

Daly, J., McDonald, I. & Willis, E. 1992, 'Why don't you ask them? A qualitative research framework for investigating the diagnosis of cardiac normality', in *Researching health care: Designs, dilemmas, disciplines*, eds J. Daly, I. McDonald & E. Willis, Routledge, London, pp. 189–206.

Davies, D. & Dodd, J. 2002, 'Qualitative research and the question of rigor', *Qualitative Health Research*, vol. 12, no. 2, pp. 279–89.

Davies, S. 2004, '"Making the move": Relatives' experiences of the transition to a care home', *Health and Social Care in the Community*, vol. 12, no. 6, pp. 517–26.

de Carvalho, M.L. 2003, 'Fathers' participation in childbirth at a public hospital: Institutional difficulties and motivations of couples', *Cad Saude Publica*, vol. 19, no. (Suppl. 2), pp. S389–98.

de Konig, K. & Martin, M. (eds) 1996, *Participatory action research in health: Issues and experiences*, Zed Books, London.

Denning, J.D. & Verschelden, C. 1993, 'Using focus groups in assessing training needs: Empowering child care workers', *Child Welfare League of America*, vol. 72, no. 6, pp. 569–79.

Denzin, N. 1970, *The research act*, Aldine, Chicago.

Denzin, N. 1989, *The research act: A theoretical introduction to sociological methods*, 3rd edn, Prentice Hall, New Jersey.

Denzin, N. 1997, *Interpretive ethnography*, Sage Publications, Thousand Oaks, California.

Denzin, N. & Lincoln, Y. 1994, *Handbook of qualitative research*, Sage Publications, Newbury Park, California.

Denzin, N. & Lincoln, Y.S. 2003, *Collecting and interpreting qualitative materials*, Sage Publications, Thousand Oaks, California.

DeSantis, G. 1980, 'Interviewing as social interaction', *Qualitative Sociology*, vol. 2, pp. 72–98.

Devers, K. 1999, 'How will we know "good" qualitative research when we see it? Beginning the dialogue in health services research', *Health Services Research*, vol. 34, no. 5, pp. 1153–88.

Devos, S.A., Baeyens, K. & Van Hecke, L. 2003, 'Suncreen use and skin protection behaviour on the Belgian beach', *International Journal of Dermatology*, vol. 42, no. 5, pp. 352–6.

Dey, I. 1993, *Qualitative data analysis: A user friendly guide for social scientists*, Routledge, London.

Dey, I. 1999, *Grounding grounded theory: Guidelines for qualitative inquiry*, Academic Press, San Diego.

Diener, E. & Crandall, R. 1978, *Ethics in social and behavioural research*, The University of Chicago Press.

Dingwall, R. & Murray, T. 1983, 'Categorisation in accident departments: "Good" patients, "bad" patients and children', *Sociology of Health and Illness*, vol. 5, pp. 127–48.

Dixon-Woods, M. & Fitzpatrick, R. 2001, 'Qualitative research in systematic reviews: Has established a place for itself', *British Medical Journal*, vol. 323, pp. 765–6.

Donner, H. 2003, 'The place of birth: Childbearing and kinship in Calcutta middle-class families', *Medical Anthropology*, vol. 22, pp. 303–41.

Douglas, J.D. 1976, *Investigative social research: Individual and team field research*, Sage Publications, Beverly Hills, California.

Dunbar, C., Rodriguez, D. & Parker, L. 2002, 'Race, subjectivity and the interview process', in *Handbook of Interview Research: Context and Method*, eds J. Gubrium & J. Holstein, Sage Publications, Thousand Oaks, California, pp. 279–98.

Easthope, C. 1997, Teachers' stories of change: An interpretive study of behavioural studies teachers' experiences of change in Tasmanian schools and colleges, PhD thesis, Deakin University.

Ellen, R.F. 1984, *Ethnographic research*, Academic Press, New York.

Ellis, C. & Bochner, A.P. 1992, 'Telling and performing personal stories: The constraints of choice in abortion', in *Investigating subjectivity: Research on lived experience*, eds C. Ellis & M. Flaherty, Sage Publications, Newbury Park, California.

Ellis, C. & Bochner A.P. 1996, *Composing ethnography: Alternative forms of qualitative writing*, AltaMira, Landham.

Emerson, R.M., Fretz, R.I. & Shaw, L.L. 1995, *Writing ethnographic fieldnotes*, University of Chicago Press.

Ezzy, D. 1998, 'Lived experience and interpretation in narrative theory', *Qualitative Sociology*, vol. 21, no. 1, pp. 169–80.

Faberman, H. 1992, 'The grounds of critique', *Symbolic Interaction*, vol. 15, no. 3, pp. 375–9.

Facey, M.E. 2003, 'The health effects of taxi driving: The case of visible minority drivers in Toronto', *Canadian Journal of Public Health*, vol. 94, no. 4, pp. 254–7.

Farran, D. 1990, 'Analysing a photograph of Marilyn Monroe', in *Feminist praxis: Research theory and epistemology in feminist sociology*, ed. L. Stanley, Routledge, London.

Fetterman, D. 1989, *Ethnography: Step by Step*, Sage Publications, Newbury Park, California.

Fielding, N.G. & Lee, R.M. 1998, *Computer analysis and qualitative research*, Sage Publications, London.

Fine, M. & Wies, L. 1998, 'Writing the "wrongs" of fieldwork: Confronting our own research/writing dilemmas in urban ethnographies', in *Being reflexive in critical educational and social research*, eds G. Shacklock & J. Smyth, Falmer Press, London.

Finlay, L. 2002, '"Outing" the researcher: The provenance, process and practice of reflexivity', *Qualitative Health Research*, vol. 12, no. 4, pp. 531–45.

Flaherty, E.G., Jones, R. & Sege, R. 2004, 'Telling their stories: Primary care pracitioners' experience evaluating and reporting injuries caused by child abuse', *Journal of Child Abuse and Neglect*, vol. 28, no. 9, pp. 939–45.

Flick, U., von Kardorff, E. & Steinke, I. 2004, 'What is qualitative research? An introduction to the field' in *A companion to qualitative research*, eds U. Flick, E. von Kardorff & I. Steinke, Sage Publications, London, pp. 3–12.

Fontana, A. & Frey, J.H. 1994, 'Interviewing: The art of science', in *Handbook of Qualitative Research*, eds N.K. Denzin & Y.S. Lincoln, Sage Publications, London, pp. 361–76.

Fontana, A. & Frey, J.H. 2003, 'The interview: From structured questions to negotiated text', in *Collecting and interpreting qualitative materials*, eds N. Denzin & Y. Lincoln, Sage Publications, Thousand Oaks, California, pp. 61–106.

Foucault, M. 1967, *Madness and civilization*, Routledge, London.

Foucault, M. 1977, *Language, counter–memory, practice*, ed. D.F. Bouchard, Cornell University Press, New York.

Foucault, M. 1980, *Power/knowledge*, Harvester Press, Brighton.

Fox, N. 1992, *The social meaning of surgery*, Open University Press, Buckingham.

Fox, N. 1993, *Postmodernism, sociology and health*, Open University Press, Buckingham.

Frank, A. 1995, *The wounded storyteller*, University of Chicago Press.

Freeman, A.C. & Sweeney, K. 2001, 'Why general practitioners do not implement evidence: Qualitative study', *British Medical Journal*, vol. 323, pp. 1100–2.

Gahnstrom-Strandqvist, K., Josephsson, S. & Tham, K. 2004, 'Stories of clients with mental illness: The structure of occupational therapists' interactions', *OTJR: Occupation, Participation and Health*, vol. 24, no. 4, pp. 134–43.

Gee, J.P. 2005, *An introduction to discourse analysis: Theory and method*, 2nd edn, Routledge, London.

Gibbs, G. 2002, *Qualitative data analysis: Explorations with NVivo*, Open University Press, London.

Gifford, S. 1996, 'Qualitative research: The soft option?' *Health Promotion Journal of Australia*, vol. 6, no. 1, pp. 58–61.

Gill, R. 1993, 'Justifying injustice: Broadcasters' accounts of inequality in radio', in *Discourse analytic research*, eds E. Burman & I. Parker, Routledge, London, pp. 75–93.

Gilliam, M.L., Warden, M., Goldstein, C. & Tapia, B. 2004, 'Concerns about contraceptive side effects among young Latinas: A focus-group approach', *Journal of Contraception*, vol. 70, no. 4, pp. 299–305.

Glaser, B. 1978, *Theoretical sensitivity*, Sociological Press, Mill Valley.

Glaser, B. & Strauss, A. 1968, *The discovery of grounded theory*, Aldine, Chicago.

Glesne, C. & Peshkin, A. 1992, *Becoming qualitative researchers*, Longman, New York.

Global Reporting Initiative, 2002, *Sustainability reporting guidelines*, Boston, www.globalreporting.org.

Goffman, E. 1961, *Asylums*, Penguin, Harmondsworth.

Grbich, C. 1999, *Qualitative research in health: An introduction*, Allen & Unwin, Sydney.

Grbich, C. & Sykes, S. 1989, *What about us? Access to school and work of young women with severe intellectuall disabilities*, Krongold Centre, Monash University, Melbourne.

Green, J. 1998, 'Commentary: Grounded theory and the constant comparative method', *British Medical Journal*, vol. 316, pp. 1064–5.

Guarnaccia, P.J. 2001, 'Introduction: The contributions of medical anthropology to anthropology and beyond', *Medical Anthropology Quarterly*, vol. 15, no. 4, pp. 423–7.

Guba, E. 1990, 'The alternative paradigm dialog', in *The paradigm dialog*, ed. E. Guba, Sage Publications, Newbury Park, California, pp. 17–30.

Guba, E. & Lincoln, Y.S. 1989, *Fourth generation evaluation*, Sage Publications, Newbury Park, California.

Guba, E. & Lincoln, Y.S. 1994, 'Competing paradigms in qualitative research', in *Handbook of qualitative research*, eds N.K. Denzin & Y.S. Lincoln, Sage Publications, Thousand Oaks, California, pp. 105–17.

Gubrium, J. & Holstein, J. 1997, *The new language of qualitative methods*, Oxford University Press, New York.

Gubrium, J. & Holstein, J. 2002, 'From the individual interview to interview society', in *Handbook of interview research: Context and method*, eds J. Gubrium & J. Holstein, Sage Publications, Thousand Oaks, California, pp. 3–32.

Hamberg, K., Johansson, E., Lindgren, G. & Westman, G. 1994, 'Scientific rigour in qualitative research – Examples from a study of women's health in family practice', *Family Practice*, vol. 11, no. 2, pp. 176–81.

Hamel, J. 2001, 'The focus group method and contemporary French sociology', *Journal of Sociology*, vol. 37, no. 4, pp. 341–54.

Hammersley, M. 1990, *Reading ethnographic research: A critical guide*, Longmans, London.

Hammersly, M. 1992, 'Deconstructing the qualitative-quantitative divide', in *Mixing methods: Qualitative and quantitative research*, ed. J. Brannen, Aldershott, Avebury.

Hammersley, M. 1993, *Educational research: Current issues*, The Open University, Paul Chapman Publishing, London.

Hammersley, M. & Atkinson, P. 1995, *Ethnography: Principles in practice*, 2nd edn, Routledge, New York.

Hansen, E.C. 2001, Medical understandings of lifestyle: An interpretive study of 'lifestyle' as a medical explanatory framework, Unpublished PhD Thesis, University of Tasmania.

Hansen, E.C. 2003, Doctors as lay epidemiologists: Areas of commonality between medical and lay accounts of lifestyle, Paper presented to *The Australian Sociological Association Conference*, University of New England.

Hansen, E.C. & Robinson, A. 2003, Identifying issues in the provision of care for people with dementia in a remote Tasmanian community, paper presented to *Australian Association of Gerontology 37th National Conference*, 12–14 November, Hobart

Hansen, E.C., Walters, J., Mudge, P., Gartlan, J., Wood Baker, R. & Walters, E.H. 2004, The Use of Spirometry by General Practitioners for the Diagnosis of Chronic Obstructive Pulmonary Disease, paper presented to *General Practice and Primary Health Research Conference: What's [not] working? How do we know?*, 2–4 June, Sheraton Hotel, Brisbane.

Hansen, E.C., Robinson, A., Mudge, P. & Crack, G. 2005, 'Barriers to the provision of care for people with dementia and their carers in a rural community', *Australian Journal of Primary Health*, vol. 11, no. 1, pp. 72–9.

Harding, G. & Gantley, M. 1998, 'Qualitative methods: Beyond the cookbook', *Family Practice*, vol. 15, pp. 76–9.

Harris, J. & Roberts, K. 2003, 'Challenging barriers to participation in qualitative research: Involving disabled refugees', *International Journal of Qualitative Methods*, vol. 2, no. 2, pp. 1–16.

Hart, E. & Bond, M. 1995, *Action research for health and social care: A guide to practice*, Open University Press, Buckingham.

Hermanowicz, J.C. 2002, 'The great interview: 25 strategies for studying people in bed', *Qualitative Sociology*, vol. 25, no. 4, pp. 479–99.

Hertz, R. & Imber, J.B. 1993, 'Fieldwork in elite settings (Introduction)', *Journal of Contemporary Ethnography*, vol. 22, no. 1, pp. 3–6.

Heyl, B.S. 2001, 'Ethnographic interviewing', in *Handbook of ethnography*, eds P. Atkinson, A. Coffey, S. Delamont, J. Lofland & L.H. Lofland, Sage Publications, London, pp. 369–83.

Hill, K. 2003, 'The sound of silence – nurses' non-verbal interaction within the ward round', *Nursing and Critical Care*, vol. 8, no. 6, pp. 231–9.

Holmstrom, I.M. & Rosenqvist, U. 2005, 'Misunderstandings about illness and treatment among patients with type 2 diabetes', *Journal of Advanced Nursing*, vol. 49, no. 2, pp. 146–54.

Holstein, J. & Gubrium, J. 1997, 'Active interviewing', in *Qualitative research: Theory, method and practice*, ed. D. Silverman, Sage Publications, London, pp. 113–29.

House, E.R. 1980, *Evaluating with validity*, Sage Publications, Beverly Hills, California.

House, E.R. 1994, 'Integrating the quantitative and qualitative', in *The quantitative-qualitative debate: New perspectives*, eds C.S. Reichardt & S.F. Rallis, Jossey-Bass, San Francisco, pp. 13–22.

Humphreys, L. 1970, *Tearoom trade: Impersonal sex in public places*, Aldine, Chicago.

Hunter, A., Lusardi, P., Zucker, D., Jacelon, C. & Chandler, G. 2002, 'Making meaning: The creative component in qualitative research', *Qualitative Health Research*, vol. 12, no. 3, pp. 388–98.

Jack, S.M., DiCenso, A. & Lohfeld, L. 2005, 'A theory of maternal engagement with public health nurses and family visitors', *Journal of Advanced Nursing*, vol. 49, no. 2, pp. 182–90.

Jain, A., Sherman, S.N., Chamberlin, L.A. & Whitaker, R.C. 2004, 'Mothers misunderstand questions on a feeding questionnaire', *Appetite*, vol. 42, no. 3, pp. 249–54.

Järviluoma, H., Moisala, P. & Vilkko, A. 2003, *Gender and qualitative methods*: *Introducing qualitative methods*, Sage Publications, London.

Jordens, C.F.C. & Little, M. 2004, '"In this scenario I do this, for these reasons": Narrative, genre and ethical reasoning in the clinic', *Social Science and Medicine*, vol. 58, no. 9, pp. 1635–45.

Kaufert, P. & O'Neill, J. 1993, 'Analysis of a dialogue on risks in childbirth: Clinicians, epidemiologists, and Inuit women', in *Knowledge, power and practice: The anthropology of medicine in everyday life*, eds S. Lindenbaum & M. Lock, University of California Press, Berkeley, pp. 32–54.

Kelle, H. 2001, 'Ethnographic methodology and problems of triangulation: The example of studies on children's peer culture', *Zeitschrift fur Soziologie der Erziehung und Socialisation*, vol. 21, no. 2, pp. 192–208.

Kelle, U. (ed.) 1995, *Computer aided qualitative data analysis: Theory, methods and practice*, Sage Publications, London.

Kelle, U. & Erzberger, C. 2004, 'Qualitative and quantitative methods: Not in opposition', in *A companion to qualitative research*, eds U. Flick, E. von Kardoff & I. Steinke, Sage Publications, London, pp. 172–7.

Kellehear, A. 1993, *The unobtrusive researcher: A guide to methods*, Allen & Unwin, Sydney.

Kemmis, S. & Wilkinson, M. 1998, 'Participatory action research and the study of practice', in *Action research in practice: Partnerships for social justice in education*, eds B. Atweh, S. Kemmis & P. Weeks, Routledge, New York, pp. 21–36.

Kimchi, J., Polivka, B. & Sabol Stevenson, J. 1991, 'Triangulation: Operational definitions', *Nursing Research*, vol. 40, no. 6, pp. 364–6.

REFERENCES

King, L., Hawe, P. & Wise, M. 1996, *From research into practice in health promotion: A review of the literature on dissemination*, Australian Centre for Health Promotion, University of Sydney.

Kirk, J. & Miller, M. 1986, *Reliability and validity in qualitative research*, Sage Publications, Newbury Park, California.

Kitzinger, J. 1990, 'Audience understanding of AIDS: A discussion of methods', *Sociology of Health and Illness*, vol. 12, pp. 319–35.

Kitzinger, J. 1994, 'The methodology of focus groups: The importance of interaction between research participants', *Sociology of Health and Illness*, vol. 16, no. 1, pp. 103–21.

Kitzinger, J. 2000, 'Focus groups with users and providers of health care', in *Qualitative research in health care*, 2nd edn, eds C. Pope & N. Mays, British Medical Journal (BMJ) Books, London.

Kleinman, A. 1988, *The illness narratives: Suffering, healing and the human condition*, Basic Books, New York.

Knafl, K.A. & Webster, D.C. 1988, 'Managing and analyzing qualitative data: A description of tasks, techniques and materials', *Western Journal of Nursing Research*, vol. 10, pp. 195–210.

Kong, T.S., Mahoney, D. & Plummer, K. 2002, 'Queering the interview', in *Handbook of interview research: Context and method*, eds J. Gubrium & J. Holstein, Sage Publications, Thousand Oaks, California, pp. 239–58.

Kotarba, J.A. 1990, 'Ethnography and AIDS: Returning to the streets', *Journal of Contemporary Ethnography*, vol. 19, no. 3, pp. 259–70.

Krippendorf, K. 1980, *Content analysis: An introduction to its methodology*, Sage Publications, London.

Krueger, R. 1994, *Focus groups: A practical guide for applied research*, 2nd edn, Sage Publications, London.

Kushman, J.W. 1992, 'The organizational dynamics of teacher workplace-place commitment: A study of urban elementary and middle schools', *Educational Administration Quarterly*, vol. 28, no. 1, pp. 5–42.

Laderman, C. 1983, *Wives and midwives: Childbirth and nutrition in rural Malaysia*, University of California Press, Berkeley.

Lambert, H. & McKevitt, C, 2002, 'Anthropology in health research: From qualitative methods to multidisciplinarity', *British Medical Journal*, vol. 325, p. 210.

Lather, P. 1988, 'Feminist perspectives on empowering research methodologies', *Women's Studies International Forum*, vol. 11, no. 6, pp. 569–81.

Lawton, J. 2001, 'Gaining and maintaining consent: Ethical concerns raised in a study of dying patients', *Qualitative Health Research*, vol. 11, no. 5, pp. 693–705.

Layder, D. 1993, *New strategies in social research: An introduction and guide*, Polity Press, Cambridge.

Lee, R.M. 2004, 'Recording technologies and the interview in sociology, 1920–2000', *Sociology*, vol. 38, no. 5, pp. 869–89.

Leininger, M. (ed.) 1985, *Qualitative research methods in nursing*, Grune & Straton, Orlando.

Leininger, M. & McFarlane, M. 2002, *Transcultural nursing: Concepts, theories, research and practice*, McGraw-Hill, New York.

Leishmann, J.L. 2003, 'Social constructionism, discourse analysis and mental health nursing: A natural synergy', *International Journal of Psychiatric Nursing Research*, vol. 9, no. 1, pp. 1004–13.

Lewis, J.M., Majoribanks, T. & Pirotta, M. 2003, 'Changing professions: General practitioners' perceptions of autonomy on the frontline', *Journal of Sociology*, vol. 39, no. 1, pp. 44–61.

Lidz, C.W. & Ricci, E.P. 1990, 'Funding large-scale qualitative sociology', *Qualitative Sociology*, vol. 13, no. 2, pp. 113–26.

Lim, L., Nathan, P., O'Brien-Malone, A. & Williams, S.T. 2004, 'A qualitative approach to identifying psychosocial issues faced by bipolar patients', *The Journal of Nervous and Mental Disease*, vol. 192, no. 12, pp. 810–17.

Lincoln, Y.S. 1992, 'Sympathetic connections between qualitative methods and health research', *Qualitative Health Research*, vol. 2, no. 4, pp. 375–91.

Lincoln, Y.S. & Guba, E. 1985, *Naturalistic inquiry*, Sage Publications, Beverly Hills, California.

Locke, L.F., Spirduso, W.W. and Silverman, S.J. 2000, *Proposals that work: A guide for planning dissertations and grant proposals*, 4th edn, Sage Publications, Thousand Oaks, California.

Loff, B. & Black, J. 2004, 'Research ethics committees: What is their contribution?', *Medical Journal of Australia*, vol. 181, no. 8, pp. 440–1.

Lofland, J. & Lofland, L.H. 1971, *Analyzing social settings*, Wadsworth, Belmont.

Lofland, J. & Lofland, L.H. 1984, *Analysing social settings*, 2nd edn, Wadsworth, Belmont.

Lofland, J. & Lofland, L.H. 1995, *Analysing social settings*, 3rd edn, Wadsworth, Belmont.

Lopez, K.A. & Willis, D.G. 2004, 'Descriptive versus interpretive phenomenology: Their contributions to nursing knowledge', *Qualitative Health Research*, vol. 14, no. 5, pp. 726–35.

Low, J.T.S., Roderick, P. & Payne, S. 2004, 'An exploration looking at the impact of domiciliary and day hospital delivery of stroke rehabilitation on informal carers', *Clinical Rehabilitation*, vol. 18, no. 7, pp. 776–84.

Lowton, K. 2004, 'Only when I cough? Adults disclosure of cystic fibrosis', *Qualitative Health Research*, vol. 14, no. 2, pp. 167–86.

Lupton, D. 1992, 'Discourse analysis: A new methodology for understanding the ideologies of health and illness', *Australian Journal of Public Health*, vol. 16, no. 2, pp. 145–9.

Lupton, D. 1994a, 'The condom in the age of AIDS: Newly respectable or still a dirty word? A discourse analysis', *Qualitative Health Research*, vol. 4, no. 3, pp. 304–20.

Lupton, D. 1994b, 'Femininity, responsibility, and the technological imperative: Discourses on breast cancer in the Australian press', *International Journal of Health Services*, vol. 24, no. 1, pp. 73–89.

Lupton, D. 1997, 'Doctors on the medical profession', *Sociology of Health and Illness*, vol. 19, pp. 480–97.

Lupton, D. & Chapman, S. 1995, 'The healthy lifestyle might be the death of you: Discourses on diet, cholesterol control and heart disease in the press and among the lay public', *Sociology of Health and Illness*, vol. 17, pp. 477–94.

REFERENCES

Lynch, M. 1993, *Scientific practice and ordinary action: Ethnomethodology and social studies of science*, Cambridge University Press, Cambridge.

McClelland, L., Reicher, S. & Booth, N. 2000, 'A last defence: The negotiation of blame within suicide notes', *Journal of Community and Applied Social Psychology*, vol. 10, no. 3, pp. 225–40.

McCracken, G. 1988, *The long interview*, Sage Publications, Newbury Park, California.

McCreigh, B.S. 2004, 'A grief ignored: Narratives of pregnancy loss from a male perspective', *Sociology of Health and Illness*, vol. 26, no. 3, pp. 326–50.

McDonald, I. & Daly, J. 1992, 'Researching methods in health care: A summing up', in *Researching health care: Designs, dilemmas, disciplines*, ed. J. Daly, I. McDonald & E. Willis, Routledge, London.

MacDougall C. & Baum, F. 1997, 'The devil's advocate: A strategy to avoid groupthink and stimulate discussion in focus groups', *Qualitative Health Research*, vol. 7, pp. 532–41.

McElroy, A. & Townsend, P.K. 1999, *Medical anthropology in ecological perspective*, 3rd edn, Macmillan Australia, South Yarra.

MacFayden, L., Amos, A., Hastings, G. & Parkes, E. 2002, '"They look like my kind of people"—perceptions of smoking images in youth magazines', *Social Science and Medicine*, vol. 56, pp. 491–9.

McKenna, L.G. & Green, C. 2004, 'Experiences and learning during a graduate nurse program: An examination using a focus group approach', *Nurse Education in Practice*, vol. 4, no. 4, pp. 258–63.

McLafferty, I. 2004, 'Focus group interviews as a data collecting strategy', *Journal of Advanced Nursing*, vol. 48, no. 2, pp. 187–94.

Macoun, A. 2004, *Working paper 2. Improving the quality of research proposals*, available at http://info.lut.ac.uk/departments/cv/wedc/garnet/actiwp2.html.

Malinowski, B. 1967, *A diary in the strict sense of the term*, Routledge, London.

Maloney, R.S. & Paolisso, M. 2001, 'What can digital audio data do for you?', *Field Methods*, vol. 13, no. 1, pp. 88–96.

Malterud, K. 1995, 'Action research – a strategy for evelution of medical interventions', *Family Practice*, vol. 12, pp. 476–81.

Manser, T., Kalucy, E., McIntyre, E., Navarro, C., Thomas, F. & Dixon, K. 2004, 'Report writing: Processes, principles and styles', *Journal Watch: Evidence-based Policy and Practice Research Bulletin*, The Primary Health Care Research and Information Service, Adelaide pp. 1–16.

Marcus, G.E. 1994, 'What comes (just) after "post"? The case of ethnography', in *Handbook of Qualitative Research*, eds N. Denzin and Y. Lincoln, Sage Publications, Newbury Park, California.

Marcus, G.E. & Fischer, M.M.J. 1986, *Anthropology as cultural critique: An experimental movement in the human sciences*, University of Chicago Press.

Mark, M.M. & Shortland, R.L. 1987, 'Alternative models for the use of multiple methods', in *Multiple methods in program evaluation: New directions for program evaluation*, eds M.M. Mark & R.L. Shortland, Jossey-Bass, San Francisco, pp. 95–100.

Martin, C.M., Banwell, C.L., Broom, D.H. & Nisa, M. 1999, 'Consultation length and chronic illness care in general practice: A qualitative study', *Medical Journal of Australia*, vol. 171, pp. 77–81.

Martin, E. 1987, *The woman in the body*, Open University Press, Milton Keynes.

Martin, J. 1994, *Action research, evaluation and health care: Widening our perspectives on nursing research*, The University of New England Press, Armidale.

Martin, P.Y. & Turner, B.A. 1986, 'Grounded theory and organisational research', *Journal of Applied Behavioural Science*, vol. 22, no. 2, pp. 141–57.

Marvasti, A.B. 2004, *Qualitative research in sociology*, Sage Publications, London.

Maxwell, J. 1996, *Qualitative research design: An interactive approach*, Sage Publications, Thousand Oaks, California.

Mayring, P. 2000, 'Qualitative content analysis [28 Paragraphs]', *Forum Qualitative Sozialforschung/ Forum: Qualitative Social Research* [on-line journal], vol. 1, no. 2.

Mays, N. & Pope, C. 2000, 'Assessing quality in qualitative research', *British Medical Journal*, vol. 320, pp. 50–2.

Mechanic, D. 1989, 'Medical sociology: Some tensions among theory, method, and substance', *Journal of Health and Social Behaviour*, vol. 30, no. 2, pp. 147–60.

Meijer, P.C., Verloop, N. & Beijaard, D. 2002, 'Multi-method triangulation in a qualitative study on teachers' practical knowledge: An attempt to increase internal validity', *Quality and Quantity*, vol. 36, no. 2, pp. 145–67.

Meloy, J. 1994, *Writing the qualitative dissertation: Understanding by doing*, Lawrence Erlbaum Associates, New Jersey.

Meredith, P. 1993, 'Patient participation in decision making and consent to treatment: The case of general surgery', *Sociology of Health and Illness*, vol. 15, no. 5, pp. 315–36.

Merton, R.K. 1956, *The focused interview*, Free Press, Glencoe.

Merriam, S.B. 1998, *Qualitative research and case study applications in education*, Jossey-Bass, San Francisco.

Mewett, P. 1989, 'Making a research topic: A continuing process', in *Doing fieldwork: Eight personal accounts of social research*, ed. J. Perry, Deakin University Printery, Geelong, pp. 73–90.

Meyer, J. 2000, 'Using qualitative methods in health-related action research', *British Medical Journal*, vol. 320, pp. 178–81.

Meyer, J. & Bridges, J. 1998, *An action research study into the organisation of care of older people in the accident and emergency department*, City University, London.

Miles, M. & Huberman, A. 1994, *Qualitative data analysis*, 2nd edn, Sage Publications, Thousand Oaks, California.

Miller, S.I. & Fredericks, M. 1996, 'Can there be "rules" for qualitative inquiry?', *Journal of Thought*, vol. 31, no. 2, pp. 61–71.

Minchiello, V., Aroni, R., Timewell, E. & Alexander, L. 1990, *In-depth interviewing: Principles, techniques, analysis*, 2nd edn, Longman Australia, Melbourne.

Mischler, E.G. 1979, 'Meaning in context: Is there any other kind?', *Harvard Educational Review*, vol. 49, no. 1, pp. 1–19.

Mischler, E.G. 1986, *Research interviewing: Context and narrative*, Harvard University Press, Cambridge, Massachusetts.

Mitchell, S.G., Peterson, J.A. & Kaya, S. 2004, 'Making the switch to digital audio', *International Journal of Qualitative Methods*, vol. 3, no. 4, retrieved 4 April 2005 from http://www.ualberta.ca/~iiqm/backissues/3_4/pdf/mitchell.pdf.

Moloney, R.S. & Paolisso, M. 2001, 'What can digital audio data do for you?', *Field Methods*, vol. 13, no. 1, pp. 88–96.

Montell, F. 1999, 'Focus group interviews: A new feminist method', *NWSA Journal*, vol. 11, pp. 44–71.

Morgan, D.L. 1997, *Focus groups as qualitative research*, 2nd edn, Sage Publications, Newbury Park, California.

Morgan, D.L. 1998, 'Practical strategies for combining qualitative and quantitative methods: Applications to health research', *Qualitative Health Research*, vol. 8, pp. 362–76.

Morison, M. & Moir, J. 1998, 'The role of computer software in the analysis of qualitative data: Efficient clerk, research assistant or Trojan horse?', *Journal of Advanced Nursing*, vol. 28, no. 1, pp. 106–16.

Morris, K., Kavanagh, A.M. & Gunn, J.M. 2001, 'Management of women with minor abnormalities of the cervix detected on screening: A qualitative study', *Medical Journal of Australia*, vol. 174, pp. 126–9.

Morse, J.M. (ed.) 1989, *Qualitative nursing research: A contemporary dialogue*, Gaithersburg, Aspen.

Morse, J.M. 1990, *Qualitative nursing research: A contemporary dialogue*, Sage Publications, Thousand Oaks, California.

Morse, J.M. 1991, 'Strategies for sampling', in *Qualitative nursing research: A contemporary dialogue*, ed. J.M. Morse, Sage Publications, Newbury Park, California, pp. 127–45.

Morse, J.M. 1994, 'Designing funded qualitative research', in *Handbook of qualitative research*, eds N.K. Denzin & Y. Lincoln, Sage Publications, Thousand Oaks, California, pp. 220–35.

Morse, J.M. 2000a, 'Editorial: Determining sample size', *Qualitative Health Research*, vol. 10, no. 1, pp. 3–5.

Morse, J.M. 2000b, 'Editorial: Theoretical congestion', *Qualitative Health Research*, vol. 10, no. 6, pp. 715–16.

Morse, J.M. & Field, P. 1995, *Qualitative research methods for health professionals*, 2nd edn, Sage Publications, Thousand Oaks, California.

Morse, J.M. & Field, P. 1996, *Nursing research: The application of qualitative approaches*, 2nd edn, Chapman & Hall, London.

Motsyn, B. 1985, 'The content analysis of qualitative research data: A dynamic approach', in *The research interview*, eds M. Brenner, J. Brown & D. Cauter, Academic Press, London, pp. 115–45.

Muhr, T. 2000, 'Increasing the reusability of qualitative data with XML', *Forum Qualitative Social Research*, vol. 1, no. 3, retrieved 4th April 2005 from http://www.qualitative-research.net/fqs-texte/3–00/3–00muhr-e.htm.

National Health and Medical Research Council 1995, *Ethical aspects of qualitative methods in health research. An information paper for institutional ethics committees*, NHMRC, Canberra.

National Health and Medical Research Council 1999, *National statement on ethical conduct in research involving humans*, Commonwealth of Australia, Canberra.

National Institute of Health: Office of Behavioural and Social Sciences Research 2005, *Qualitative methods in health research: Opportunities and considerations in application and review*, online report downloaded 21 April 2005 from http://www.obssr.od.nih.gov/Publications/Qualitative.PDF.

National Institute on Disability and Rehabilitation Research 2001, *Developing an effective dissemination plan*, Southwest Educational Development Laboratory, available at http://www.ncddr.org/du/products/dissplan.html.

Nettleton, S. 1991, 'Wisdom, diligence and teeth: Discursive practices and the creation of mothers', *Sociology of Health and Illness*, vol. 13, no. 1, pp. 98–111.

Nettleton, S. 1992, *Power, pain and dentistry*, McGraw-Hill, London.

Nettleton, S. 1995, *The sociology of health and illness*, Polity Press, Cambridge.

Neuman, W.L. 1994, *Social research methods: Qualitative and quantitative approaches*, Allyn & Bacon, Boston.

Neuman, W.L. 2000, *Social research methods: Qualitative and quantitative approaches*, 4th edn, Allyn & Bacon, Boston.

Nichter, M., Nichter, M., Vukovick, N., Teslter, L., Adrian, S. & Ritenbaugh, C. 2004, 'Smoking as a weight-control strategy among adolescent girls and young women: A reconsideration, *Medical Anthropology Quarterly*, vol. 18, no. 3, pp. 305–24.

Nucifora, A. 2000, 'Internet is revolutionizing the use of focus groups', *Orlando Business Journal*, vol. 17, no. 17, p. 49.

Nunan, D. 1993, *Introducing discourse analysis*, Penguin, Harmondsworth.

Oakley, A. 1981, 'Interviewing women: A contradiction in terms?', in *Doing feminist research*, ed. H.E. Roberts, Routledge & Kegan Paul, London, pp. 30–61.

O'Brian, R. 1998, *An overview of the methodological approach of action research*, available at http://www.web.net/~robrian/papers/arfinal.html.

O'Brien, K. 1993, 'Improving survey questionnaires through focus groups', in *Successful focus groups: Advancing the state of the art*, ed. D.L. Morgan, Sage Publications, London, pp. 105–18.

Oiler Boyd, C. 1993, 'Towards a nursing practice research method', *Advanced Nursing Science*, vol. 16, no. 2, pp. 9–25.

Ong, E.K. & Glantz, S.A. 2001, 'Constructing "sound science" and "good epidemiology": Tobacco lawyers and public relations firms', *American Journal of Public Health*, vol. 91, no. 11, pp. 1749–57.

Ovretveit, J. 1998, *Evaluating health interventions: An introduction to evaluation of health treatments, services, policies and organizational interventions*, Open University Press, Buckingham and Philadelphia.

Owen, J.M. & Rogers, P.J. 1999, *Program evaluation: Forms and approaches*, 2nd edn, Allen & Unwin, Sydney.

Parker, I. 1992, *Discourse dynamics: Critical analysis for social and individual psychology*, Routledge, London.

Parry, O., Fowkes, F.G.R. & Thompson, C. 2001, 'Accounts of quitting among older ex-smokers with smoking-related disease', *Journal of Health Psychology*, vol. 6, no. 5, pp. 481–93.

Patton, M.Q. 1990, *Qualitative evaluation and research methods*, 2nd edn, Sage Publications, Newbury Park, California.

Patton, M.Q. 1997, *Utilization focused evaluation: The new century text*, 3rd edn, Sage Publications, Newbury Park, California.

Patton, M.Q. 1999, 'Enhancing the quality and credibility of qualitative analysis', *Health Services Research*, vol. 34, no. 5, pp. 1189–208.

Perry, J. (ed.) 1989, *Doing fieldwork: Eight personal accounts of social research*, Deakon University Press, Geelong.

Plumridge, E.W., Fitzgerald, L.J. & Abel, G.M. 2002, 'Performing coolness: Smoking refusal and adolescent identities', *Health Education Research*, vol. 17, no. 2, pp. 167–79.

Popay, J., Williams, G. & Rogers, A. 1998, 'Rationale and standards for the systematic review of qualitative literature in health services research', *Qualitative Health Research*, vol. 8, pp. 341–51.

Pope, C. & Mays, N. (eds) 1995a, *Qualitative research in health care*, British Medical Journal (BMJ) Books, London.

Pope, C. & Mays, N. 1995b, 'Researching the parts other methods cannot reach: An introduction to qualitative methods in health and health services research', *British Medical Journal*, vol. 311, pp. 42–5.

Pope, C. & Mays, N. (eds) 2000, *Qualitative research in health care*, 2nd edn, British Medical Journal (BMJ) Books, London.

Pope, C., Ziebland, S. & Mays, N. 2000, 'Analysing qualitative data', *British Medical Journal*, vol. 320, pp. 114–16.

Potter, J. & Wetherell, M. 1987, *Discourse and social psychology*, Sage Publications, London.

Power, R., Jones, S., Kearns, G. & Ward, J. 1996, 'An ethnography of risk management amongst illicit drug injectors and its implications for the development of community based interventions', *Sociology of Health and Illness*, vol. 18, no. 1, pp. 89–106.

Prus, R. 1996, *Symbolic interaction and ethnographic research*, State University of New York Press, Albany.

Pryke, M., Rose, G. & Whatmore, S.E. 2003, *Using social theory: Thinking through research*, Sage Publications, London.

Punch, K.E. 1998, *Introduction to social research: Quantitative and qualitative approaches*, Sage Publications, London.

Punch, M. 1986, *The politics and ethics of fieldwork*, Sage Publications, New Delhi.

QSR 2002, *NVivo: Using NVivo in qualitative research*, QSR International, Melbourne.

Rapp, R. 1988, 'Chromosomes and communication: The discourse of genetic counselling', *Medical Anthropology Quarterly*, vol. 2, pp. 143–57.

Rice, P.L. 1996, 'Health research and ethnic communities: Reflection on practice', in *Health Research in Practice, Volume 2: Personal Experiences, Public Issues*, eds D. Colquhoun & A. Kellehear, Chapman & Hall, London.

Rice, P.L. & Ezzy, D. 1999, *Qualitative research methods: A health focus*, Oxford University Press, Melbourne.

Richards, H. & Emslie, C. 2000, 'The "doctor" or the "girl from the university"?

Considering the influence of professional roles on qualitative interviewing', *Family Practice*, vol. 17, no. 1, pp. 71–5.

Richards, H.M. & Schwartz, L.J. 2002, 'Ethics of qualitative research: Are there special issues for health services research?', *Family Practice*, vol. 19, no. 2, pp. 135–9.

Richardson, L. 1990, *Writing strategies: Reaching diverse audiences*, Sage Publications, Newbury Park, California.

Richardson, L. 1991, 'Postmodern social theory: Representational practices', *Social Theory*, vol. 9, pp. 173–9.

Richardson, L. 2003, 'Writing: A method of inquiry', in *Collecting and interpreting qualitative materials*, 2nd edn, eds N. Denzin & Y. Lincoln, Sage Publications, Thousand Oaks, California, pp. 499–541.

Riessman, C.K. 1993, *Narrative analysis*, Sage Publications, Newbury Park, California.

Ritchie, J. 2001, 'Not everything can be reduced to numbers', in *Health Research*, ed. C.A. Berglund, Oxford University Press, Oxford, pp. 149–73.

Roberts, H.E. 1989, *Doing feminist research*, Routledge & Kegan Paul, London.

Roberts, K. & Taylor, B. 1998, *Nursing research process: An Australian perspective*, International Thompson Publishing Co., Melbourne.

Ronai, C. 1992, 'The reflexive self through narrative: A night in the life of an erotic dancer/researcher', in *Investigating subjectivity: Research on lived experience*, eds C. Ellis & M. Flaherty, Sage Publications, Newbury Park, California.

Rosenthal, G. 2003, 'The healing effects of storytelling: On the conditions of curative storytelling in the context of research and counselling', *Qualitative Inquiry*, vol. 9, no. 6, pp. 915–33.

Roulston, K., deMarrais, K. & Lewis, J.B. 2003, 'Learning to interview in the social sciences', *Qualitative Inquiry*, vol. 9, no. 4, pp. 643–68.

Rowan, M. & Huston, P. 1997, 'Qualitative research articles: Information for authors and peer reviewers', *Canadian Medical Association Journal*, vol. 157, pp. 1442–5.

Royse, D., Thyer, B.A., Padgett, D.K. & Logan, T.K. 2001, *Programme evaluation: An introduction*, 3rd edn, Wadsworth Books/ Cole Social Work, Belmont.

Rubin, H.J. & Rubin, I.S. 1995, *Qualitative interviewing: The art of hearing data*, Sage Publications, Thousand Oaks, California.

Rubin, R. 2004, 'Men talking about viagra: An exploratory story with focus groups', *Men and Masculinities*, vol. 7, no. 1, pp. 22–30.

Ruckdeschel, R., Earnshaw, P. & Firrek, A. 1994, 'The qualitative case study and evaluation: Issues, methods and examples', in *Qualitative Research in Social Work*, eds E. Sherman & W.J. Reid, Columbia University Press, New York.

Sacks, V. 1996, 'Women and AIDS: An analysis of media misrepresentations', *Social Science and Medicine*, vol. 42, no. 1, pp. 59–73.

Sale, J.E.M., Lohfeld, L.H. & Brazil, K. 2002, 'Revisiting the quantitative-qualitative debate: Implications for mixed-methods research', *Quality and Quantity*, vol. 36, pp. 43–53.

Sandelowski, M. 1993, 'Rigor or rigor-mortis – The problem of rigor in qualitative research revisited', *Advances In Nursing Science*, vol. 16, no. 2, pp. 1–8.

Sandelowski, M. 1995, 'Focus on qualitative methods: Sample size in qualitative research', *Research in Nursing and Health*, vol. 18, pp. 179–83.

Sanjek, R. (ed.) 1990, *Fieldnotes: The making of anthropology*, Cornell University Press, New York.

Sayre, J. 2000, 'The patient's diagnosis: Explanatory models of mental illness', *Qualitative Health Research*, vol. 10, no. 1, pp. 71–83.

Schatzman, L. & Strauss, A. 1973, *Field research: Strategies for a natural sociology*, Prentice Hall, Englewood Cliffs.

Schutz, A. 1967, *The phenomenology of the social world*, Northwestern University Press, Chicago.

Schutz, A. 1971, 'The stranger: An essay in social psychology', in *Alfred Schutz: Collected papers II: The problem of social reality*, ed. A. Broderson, Martinus Nijohoff, The Hague, pp. 99–117.

Scott, D.A., Valery, P.C., Boyl, F.M. & Bain, C.J. 2002, 'Does research into sensitive areas do harm? Experiences of research participation after a child's diagnosis with Ewing's sarcoma', *Medical Journal of Australia*, no. 177, November, pp. 507–10.

Seale, C. 1999, 'Quality in qualitative research', *Qualitative Inquiry*, vol. 5, no. 4, pp. 465–78.

Seidel, J. 1991, 'Method and madness in the application of computer technology to qualitative data analysis', in *Using computers in qualitative research*, eds N.G. Fielding & R.M. Lee, Sage Publications, London, pp. 107–16.

Seidel, J., Freise, S. & Leonard, D.C. 1995, *The ethnograph V4.0tm: A users guide*, Quails Research Associated, Amherst, Massachusetts.

Seidman, I. 1998, *Interviewing as qualitative research: A guide for researchers in education and the social sciences*, 2nd edn, Teachers College Press, New York.

Seymour, J., Gott, M., Bellamy, G., Ahmedzai, S.H. & Clark, D. 2004, 'Planning for the end of life: The views of older people about advance care statements', *Social Science and Medicine*, vol. 59, no. 1, pp. 57–68.

Shacklock, G. & Smyth, J. (eds) 1998, *Being reflexive in critical educational and social research*, Falmer Press, Taylor & Francis Inc, London.

Shadish, W.R., Cook, T.C. & Leviton, L.C. 1991, *Foundations of program evaluation: Theories of practice*, Sage Publications, Thousand Oaks, California.

Shelby, R.D. 2000, 'Using the mentoring relationship to facilitate rigor in qualitative research', *Smith College Studies in Social Work*, vol. 70, no. 2, pp. 315–27.

Shepard, K.F., Hack, L.M., Gwyer, J. & Jensen, G.M. 1999, 'Describing expert practice in physical therapy', *Qualitative Health Research*, vol. 9, no. 6, pp. 746–58.

Sieber, J.E. 1998, 'Planning ethically responsible research', in *Handbook of applied social research methods*, eds L. Bickman & D.J. Rog, Sage Publications, Thousand Oaks, California, pp. 127–56.

Silbey, S.S. 2003, *Designing qualitative research projects*, available at: http://web.mit.edu/anthropology/faculty_staff/silbey/pdf/49DesigningQualRes.doc.

Silverman, D. 1997, *Qualitative research: Theory, method and practice*, Sage Publications, London.

Silverman, D. 2001, *Interpreting qualitative data: Methods for analyzing talk, text and interaction*, Sage Publications, London.

Silverman, D. 2003, 'Analyzing talk and text', in *Collecting and interpreting qualitative materials*, 2nd edn, eds N.K. Denzin & Y.S. Lincoln, Sage Publications, Thousand Oaks, California, pp. 340–62.

Smith, D. 1987, *The everyday world as problematic: A feminist sociology*, Open University Press, Milton Keynes.

Smith, M.L. & Glass, G.V. 1987, *Research and evaluation in education and the social sciences*, Prentice-Hall, Englewood Cliffs.

Snadden, D. 2001, 'Qualitative methods and guideline implementation – a heady mixture?', *Medical Education*, vol. 35, no. 12, pp. 1099–100.

Sofaer, S. 1999, 'Qualitative methods: What are they and why use them?', *Health Services Research*, vol. 34, no. 2, pp. 461–83.

Spencer, G. 1991, 'Methodological issues in the study of bureaucratic elites: A case study of West Point', in *Field research: A sourcebook and field manual*, ed. R.G. Burgess, Routledge, New York.

Spradley, J.P. 1970, *You owe yourself a drunk: An ethnography of urban nomads*, Little, Brown, Boston.

Spradely, J.P. 1979, *The ethnographic interview*, Reinhardt & Winston, Holt USA.

Stewart, D.W. & Shamdasani, P.N. 1990, *Focus groups: Theory and practice*, Sage Publications, Newbury Park, California.

Stockdale, A. 2000, 'Tools for digital recording in qualitative research', *Sociology at Surrey: Social research update Autumn 2002*, Published quarterly by the Department of Sociology, University of Surrey, retrieved 4 April 2005 from http://www.soc.surrey.ac.uk/sru/SRU38.html.

Stone, L. & Campbell, J.G. 1986, 'The use and misuse of surveys in international development: An experiment from Nepal', *Human Organisation*, vol. 43, pp. 27–37.

Strauss, A. & Corbin, J. 1990, *Basics of qualitative research: Grounded theory procedures and techniques*, Sage Publications, Newbury Park, California.

Strauss, A. & Corbin, J. 1994, 'Grounded theory methodology: An overview', in *Handbook of qualitative research*, N.K. Denzin & Y.S. Lincoln, eds, Sage Publications, Newbury Park, California.

Sussman, S., Burton, D., Dent, C.W., Stacey, A.W. & Flay, B.R. 1991, 'The use of focus groups in developing an adolescent tobacco use cessation program: Collection norm effects', *Journal of Applied Social Psychology*, vol. 21, pp. 1772–82.

Taft, L. 1993, 'Computer assisted qualitative research', *Research in Nursing and Health*, vol. 16, no. 5, pp. 379–83.

Tashakkori, A. & Teddlie, C. (eds), 2003, *Handbook of mixed methods in the social and behavioural sciences*, Sage Publications, Thousand Oaks, California.

Taylor, S. & Bogdan, R. 1998, *Introduction to qualitative research methods*, John Wiley & Sons, New York.

Tesch, R. 1990, *Qualitative research: Analysis types and software tools*, Falmer Press, New York.

Thomas, C., Morris, S.M. & Clark, D. 2004, 'Place of death: Preferences among cancer patients and their carers', *Social Science and Medicine*, vol. 58, no. 12, pp. 2431–44.

Thomas, J., Harden, A., Oakley, A., Oliver, S., Sutclife, K, Rees, R., Brunton, G. & Kavanagh, J. 2004, 'Integrating qualitative research with trials in systematic reviews', *British Medical Journal*, vol. 328, pp. 1010–12.

Thompson, B. 1995, 'Ethical dimensions in trauma research', *American Sociologist*, vol. 26, no. 2, pp. 54–69.

Travers, M. 2001, *Qualitative research through case studies*, Sage Publications, London.

Tulelli, S. 2003, 'Methodological triangulation and empirical research: The contribution of Paul F. Lazarsfeld', *Sociologiae Ricerca Sociale*, vol. 24, no. 72, pp. 37–61.

Tulloch, J. & Chapman, S. 1992, 'Experts in crisis: The framing of radio debate about the risk of AIDS to heterosexuals', *Discourse and Society*, vol. 3, pp. 437–67.

Ueland, B. 1991, *If you want to write: Releasing your creative spirits*, Shaftesbury, Dorset.

Vallance, R.J. 2001, 'Gaining access: Introducing refereed approval', *Issues in Educational Research*, vol. 11, pp. 65–73.

Varcoe, C., Rodney, P. & McCormick, J. 2003, 'Healthcare relationships in context: An analysis of three ethnographies', *Qualitative Health Research*, vol. 13, no. 7, pp. 957–73.

Vidich, A.J. & Lyman, S.M. 1994, 'Qualitative methods: Their history in sociology and anthropology', in *Handbook of qualitative research*, eds N. Denzin & Y. Lincoln, Sage Publications, London, pp. 23–59.

Wager, K.A., Wickham, F., Bradford, W.D., Jones, W. & Kilpatrick, A.O. 2004, 'Qualitative evaluation of South Carolina's postpartum/infant home visit program', *Public Health Nursing*, vol. 21, no. 6, pp. 541–6.

Waitzkin, H., Britt, T. & Williams, C. 1994, 'Narratives of ageing and social problems in medical encounters with older persons', *Journal of Health and Social Behaviour*, vol. 35, no. 322–48.

Walters, J.A.E., Hansen, E., Mudge, P., Johns, D.P., Walters, E.H. & Wood-Baker, R. 2005, 'Barriers to the use of spirometry in general practice', *Australian Family Physician*, vol. 34, no. 3, pp. 201–3.

Ward, J. & Holman, D. 2001, 'Who needs to plan?', in *Health Research*, ed. C.A. Berglund, Oxford University Press, London, pp. 47–62.

Warren, C.B. 1977, 'Fieldwork in the gay world: Issues in phenomenological research', *Journal of Social Issues*, vol. 33, no. 4, pp. 93–105.

Warren, C.B., Barnes-Brus, T., Burgess, H., Wiebold-Lippisch, L., Hackney, J., Harkness, G., Kennedy, V., Dingwall, R., Rosenblatt, P.C., Ryen, A. & Shuy, R. 2003, 'After the interview', *Qualitative Sociology*, vol. 26, no. 1, pp. 93–110.

Wax, R. 1960, 'Twelve years later: An analysis of field experiences', in *Human Organisational Research: Field relations and techniques*, eds R.N. Adams & J.J. Preiss, Dorsey, Homewood, pp. 166–78.

Weitzman, E.A. 1999, 'Analyzing qualitative data with computer software', *Health Services Research*, vol. 34, no. 5, pp. 1241–63.

Wellings, K., Field, J., Johnson, A. & Wadsworth, J. 1994, *Sexual behaviour in Britain: The national survey of sexual attitudes and lifestyles*, Penguin, Harmondsworth.

Wenger, G.C. 2001, 'Interviewing older people', in *Handbook of interview research*, eds J. Gubrium & J. Holstein, Sage Publications, Thousand Oaks, California, pp. 259–78.

Whittaker, A. 1996, 'Qualitative methods in general practice research: Experience from the Oceanpoint study', *Family Practice*, vol. 13, pp. 310–16.

Whitworth, J. 1994, 'The direction of medical research in Australia', *Collegian*, vol. 1, no. 1, pp. 26–8.

Whyte, W.F. 1982, 'Interviewing in field research', in *Field research: A sourcebook and field manual*, ed. R.G. Burgess, George Allen & Unwin, London, pp. 111–22.

Williams, G. 1984, 'The genesis of chronic illness: Narrative reconstruction', *Sociology of Health and Illness*, vol. 6, no. 2, pp. 175–200.

Wilson, C.S. 1973, 'Food taboos of childbirth: The Malay example', *Ecology of Food and Nutrition*, vol. 2, pp. 267–74.

Wolcott, H.F. 2001, *Writing up qualitative research*, 2nd edn, Sage Publications, Thousand Oaks, California.

Zeitlyn, S. & Rowshan, R. 1997, 'Privileged knowledge and mothers' "perceptions": The case of breast-feeding and insufficient milk in Bangladesh', *Medical Anthropology Quarterly*, vol. 11, no. 1, pp. 56–68.

INDEX